Y0-BDA-787

# LAWRENCE LITWACK, A.B., M.A., Ed.D.

Professor and Chairman, Department of Counseling
and Personnel Services Education, Kent State
University, Kent, Ohio

# ROBERT SAKATA, A.B., M.A., Ph.D.

Assistant Professor, Department of Counseling and
Personnel Services Education, and Director,
Guidance Bureau, Kent State University, Kent, Ohio

# MAY WYKLE, R.N., B.S., M.S.

Assistant Professor, Psychiatric Nursing, Frances
Payne Bolton School of Nursing, Case-Western
Reserve University, Cleveland, Ohio

# *Counseling, Evaluation and Student Development in Nursing Education*

5657

*1972*

W. B. SAUNDERS COMPANY

PHILADELPHIA · LONDON · TORONTO

W. B. Saunders Company:  West Washington Square
Philadelphia, Pa. 19105

12 Dyott Street
London, WC1A 1DB

833 Oxford Street
Toronto 18, Ontario

Counseling, Evaluation and Student Development in          ISBN 0-7216-5789-3
Nursing Education

Print No.:     9     8     7     6     5     4     3     2     1

# *Preface*

The ideas presented in this book are designed to meet the needs of nursing educators at all levels. It is our firm belief that counseling is a generic base—that the ability to form human relationships in a helping manner is not a talent unique to any profession. It is true that problems and resources available may differ from situation to situation. Nevertheless, the basic ingredients in counseling as a helping relationship remain relatively constant.

This book is dedicated to the countless numbers of professionals in the field of nursing education. By professionals, we refer to those persons who constantly strive to improve themselves and their profession, who are receptive to new ideas and approaches, and who welcome the contributions from others in allied health fields such as psychology, sociology, education, and counseling. It is our hope that this book will facilitate the development of these professionals and assist them to grow in their leadership positions in nursing education. In other words, it is dedicated to those who are committed to nursing education.

We would like to express our appreciation to those nursing educators who assisted in the research phase of this book. We refer specifically to Nancy Geisser, Alice Gorton, Barbara Gruber, Helen Kreigh, Edith Pence, Jo Ann Robinette, and Ruth Switzer. We would also like to thank Helen Ludwig, R.N., for her excellent research work, George Lucht and Donald Wonderly, who contributed ideas for Part 2 on evaluation, Kevin Coleman, who contributed material on drug counseling and on death and dying, and Tom Haenle, who contributed the chapter on student development. Special thanks go to Betty Reid and Becky Snyder for the typing of the manuscript. We are deeply grateful to all—without their assistance and support, our task would have been more difficult.

With this brief preface, we present this book, not with the thought that the ideas incorporated here represent universal truths but rather that they may serve as stimuli to the development of new and better ways of doing what we try to do.

MAY WYKLE
ROBERT SAKATA
LAWRENCE LITWACK

# Introduction

In beginning a work of this sort the reader may logically ask why such a book was written. Perhaps the simplest answer lies in several underlying assumptions, which, though fundamental, are by no means universally accepted. These assumptions, and their rationale, represent the *raison d'être* for this book. They may be stated as follows:

1. As institutions of higher education, whether alone or part of a larger system, schools of nursing have students with the same needs, problems, and concerns as those in any other group of institutions of higher education. This means that the guidance and counseling model used in public schools is inappropriate for schools of nursing. Students of nursing have not only the same concerns as other men and women their age in colleges and universities, but also many additional unique concerns which force them to learn and mature much more quickly than their peers outside of nursing. It also means that faculty members in schools of nursing may need to develop much greater skill in working directly with students, and learn to utilize referral resources when appropriate both from within and outside the school.

2. We assume that the faculty in schools of nursing do an excellent job of educating their students to become highly skilled nurses. Yet the problems inherent in trying to meet the personal-social needs of students, and in trying to develop some valid and reliable assessment tools to measure a student's progress, have continued to plague nursing educators. Many faculty members who are totally dedicated to working closely with students find themselves handicapped by the lack of readily accessible resource material in the above-mentioned areas. As the students we recruit into the profession of nursing become more diverse, so will we need to develop new and better methods of reconciling their needs with the needs of the profession.

## COUNSELING AND THE NURSE-PATIENT RELATIONSHIP

In recent years there have been innumerable references in nursing literature to the new role of the nurse. Although at times this role may become somewhat ambiguous in practice, the nurse today is expected to provide competent, safe total care for each patient for whom she has responsibility. In addition to fulfilling her historic role of providing physical care for the patient, the nurse is increasingly being asked to assume some of the functions normally fulfilled by a counselor, therapist or social worker. If we are to expect the nurse to fulfill these new roles, then there is a need to provide the additional necessary skills and understanding. For example, the nurse who will function as a community change agent emphasizing preventive health care will need a much deeper understanding of sociological principles than will the nurse who will be functioning with a primary emphasis on treatment and patient care.

Schools of nursing provide some form of training in communication skills. This training should be provided in greater collaboration with experts in the fields of communication skills, counseling, psychology, and others. It is our firm belief that the ability to form close, human, helping relationships is a necessary characteristic in nursing and other helping professions. Perhaps an ideal educational pattern would be to merge programs in nursing and the allied health professions into a comprehensive department or college of behavioral studies and services. It is, of course, true that each profession requires certain unique skills and techniques. If these skills and techniques are learned in a vacuum, however, i.e. without any real understanding of the inherent relationships with other professions, then we may be doing little more than producing competent technicians within each field. If our hope is to produce creative, talented nurses who care deeply about others, and who wish to strive constantly for new and better ways to do their jobs, then we need to re-examine our educational patterns and practices.

Faculty members tend to be highly skilled, highly trained people in their professional areas, but many have had inadequate preparation in measurement and evaluation, sound teaching techniques, or in counseling and advising students in ways more helpful to all concerned. In many ways we are describing a holistic, integrated approach to meeting the needs of our students. The better we can prepare faculty members to fulfill their educative, remedial, and guidance functions, and the more support services we can provide, the better we may be able to deal with student concerns, and the more we may be able to lower or eliminate educational barriers to learning.

## COUNSELING AND EVALUATION

Normally, in any discussion of guidance, counseling, and personnel services, the entire area of measurement and evaluation is either absent or is treated in terms of evaluation tools used for diagnostic purposes. For example, the questions of selected criteria for admission to schools of nursing, paper-and-pencil group tests used for guidance and self-understanding, and the use of standardized tests in nursing education all need to be examined in the light of current practices and possible future applications.

The area of classroom and clinical evaluation also needs to be emphasized. The way such an assessment program is planned, implemented, and evaluated can have a profound effect on the ongoing process of nursing education and on the qualities demonstrated by the graduates of a particular school, and, most important in terms of inclusion in this book, can greatly influence the success or failure of a counseling and student personnel program. If such evaluation is done primarily to determine who remains and who is dismissed, then the climate in the school tends to be one of confusion in students' minds, fear of faculty reprisal through grades, and the creation of emotional barriers to learning.

On the other hand, if such evaluation is done fairly and as objectively as possible, if the emphasis is upon the diagnosis of individual student progress for the purpose of planning remedial work, and if it is used as a teaching and learning tool planned cooperatively with students, then such a system of measurement and evaluation can contribute greatly to student growth and development. Most important, it can contribute greatly to an atmosphere of mutual respect and trust between faculty and students that creates an ideal climate for learning. Therefore it is important in any discussion of counseling and the student personnel program to look also at evaluation practices and principles.

## COUNSELING AND THE STUDENT PERSONNEL PROGRAM

Throughout our discussion of counseling services it must be remembered that the tools and skill of counseling are really means to an end—the end being to assist a student through a helping relationship to maximize his ability to live a healthy, happy, self-fulfilling life in as complete a manner as possible. As such, counseling services take their place as part of a larger picture. Counseling, whether individual or group, is a part of guidance, a process which seeks to assist the student in a variety of ways. Guidance services are also part of a larger picture, that being the broad student personnel services program within each institution of higher education.

Within the framework of student personnel may be found a number of important areas. These include student housing, student government, admissions and records, orientation programs, and guidance and counseling. The inclusion of student personnel services in this book is based on the realization that guidance and counseling services cannot exist alone. The success of any counseling program depends to a large extent on its place as part of a comprehensive student personnel program and philosophy. A well-planned and im-plemented student personnel program will lessen the need for counseling services by serving a preventive function within the in-stitution. Counseling alone, without such an integrated program, may tend to be primarily crisis-oriented, a stopgap emergency measure.

## SUMMARY

This introduction is designed to outline the rationale that served as the cornerstone in planning the organization of this book. It should be emphasized from the outset that the ideas presented here relating to counseling, evaluation, and student personnel services are not viewed as panaceas for all problems in a nursing educational system. Nor are they intended to serve as a straitjacket to make faculty members conform in a standardized manner to the demands and pressures of the educational system in which they find themselves. A good educational system, including counseling, evaluation, and student services, can exist only in a climate of security and mutual trust be-tween and among faculty members and student nurses. The higher the level of trust, the less threatening the educational atmosphere, and the greater the mutual commitment to learning by faculty and students, the greater the learning and progress of each student nurse.

It should be obvious that we are committed to a dynamic form of education within schools of nursing. We believe in faculty and students working together in the most meaningful and productive manner possible. We believe in an open, cooperative, individually self-fulfilling nursing education program designed to produce the kind of nurse who comes much closer to our ideal. We believe in a faculty, a curriculum, teaching methods, and a student services program that are continually evaluated in terms of assistance or hindrance for students moving through our nursing educational program. This philosophy represents the foundation upon which many of the ideas presented in this book rest quite firmly.

# Contents

Part 1

*Counseling*

Chapter 1

*Counseling: A Base of Operations*                3

  What Is Counseling?                          3
    *Interviewing*                           5
    *Advising*                               5
    *Supporting*                             6
    *Guiding*                                7
    *Counseling*                             8
  Why Counsel?                                 9
  When to Counsel                             10
  Bringing the Student In                     11
  Summary                                     12

Chapter 2

*Counseling and the Helping Relationship*        13

  Principles of Counseling                    13
  Ethical Standards of Counseling             15
  Characteristics of the Counselor            18
  The Core of the Helping Relationship        20
  The Counselor, the Teacher, and the Nurse   22
  Counseling: Who Does It?                    23

Chapter 3

*The Counseling Session*                                               29

    How Counseling Begins                                    29
    The Kind of Contact                                      32
    Before the Session Begins                                34
    Opening the Counseling Session                           36
    During the Counseling Session                            38
    Closing the Counseling Session                           40
    Following the Session                                     41
    Summary                                                  42


Chapter 4

*Counselee Needs and Concerns*                                         43

    Who Should Be Counseled                                  43
    Drugs and the Nursing Student                            45
      *Identification of Drug Abuse*                     48
      *Emergency Care for Drug Abuse*                    49
      *Professional Concerns About Drug Abuse*           50
    Problems in the Counseling Relationship                  52


Chapter 5

*Special Concerns of the Nursing Student*                              56

    Individuality and the Role of the Nurse                  56
    Sexuality and Nursing                                    57
    Sex Education                                            57
    Men in Nursing                                           58
    Abortion                                                 60
    Acceptance of Loss                                       62
    The Nursing Student and the Dying Patient                62
    The Culturally Different Student                         70
    The Older Student                                        72
    Summary                                                  73


Chapter 6

*Group Approaches to Guidance and Counseling*                          74

    Orientation Programs                                     74
    Vocational Group Guidance in Nursing Education           77
    Educational Group Guidance in Nursing Education          79
    Group Counseling in Nursing Education                    81
    Sensitivity Groups in Schools of Nursing                 86

Chapter 7

*Use of Referral Resources*

90

When to Refer                                    90
Referral to Whom?                                92
How to Refer                                     96
Some General Observations                        97
Bibliography (Part 1)                           100

Part 2

*Evaluation*

Chapter 8

*Introduction to Measurement*

105

Educational and Behavioral Objectives           105
Measurement                                     108
  *Role of Measurement*                         108
  *Scales*                                      109
  *Symbols and Definitions*                     110
  *Scores*                                      110
  *The Normal Curve*                            111
  *Normal Distribution*                         112
  *Percentiles*                                 113
  *Percentile Rank*                             113
  *Measures of Centralness*                     113
  *Mean and Standard Deviation*                 114
  *Standard Scores*                             115
  *Stanines*                                    116
Correlation                                     116
Standardized Measurement                        117
  *Validity*                                    117
  *Reliability*                                 118
  *Norm*                                        118
  *Usability*                                   118
Grading                                         119

Chapter 9

*Construction of Classroom Tests*

121

Frame of Reference for Test Construction        121
Some General Considerations                     123
The Objective Examination                       124
  *Completion Test Items*                       124
  *Multiple-Choice Items*                       126

*True-False or Alternative-Answer Items*                          128
*Matching-Test Items*                                             129
*Classification-Test Items*                                       130
*Identification-Test Items*                                       131
*Listings or Enumeration-Test Items*                              131
The Correction for Guessing                                       132
Item Analysis                                                     133
Essay Examinations                                                134
Situation or Problem-Solving Examinations                         137
Other Factors to Be Considered in Test Construction               138
Summary                                                           138


Chapter 10

*Clinical Evaluation*                                             141


The Qualification Process                                         142
Minimal Competency and Desirable Performance                      143
Feedback and the Qualification Process                            144
Simulated Learning                                                147
Selection of Learning Activities                                  148
Methods of Supervision                                            149
Audiovisual Aids                                                  152
Instructor Reports                                                153
Rating Scales                                                     155
Check Lists and Other Tools                                       157
Self-Ratings and Peer Ratings                                     159
Evaluation Conferences                                            160
Bibliography (Part 2)                                             161


Part 3

*Student Development*

Chapter 11

*Standardized Tests*                                              167


Pre-Entrance Tests                                                167
Placement Tests                                                   171
Achievement Tests                                                 172
Prediction of State Board Scores                                  175
State Board Licensure Examinations                                176
Studies of the Nursing Student                                    178
Tests for Guidance                                                179
Overview of Standardized Tests                                    180


Chapter 12

*Admissions and Records*                                          182


Admission Criteria                                                182
*Personal Characteristics*                                        183

Academic Achievement                                                183
Required Courses                                                    184
Personality and Vocational Interests                               184
Health Requirements                                                184
Recommendations                                                    184
Preadmission Interview                                             185
Recruitment                                                         186
Who Is Responsible for Recruitment?                                186
Recruitment Methods                                               187
Student Records                                                     191
Student Recommendations                                             192

Chapter 13

*Attrition in Schools of Nursing*                                193

Attrition Studies                                                   193
Predicting Success in Nursing Programs                              195
Prenursing and Guidance Examination                            195
SAT-ACT-GPA                                                         196
Personality, Attitude, and Interest Tests as Predictors of Success   197
Combined Predictors of Success in Nursing                           199
Conclusions                                                         201

Chapter 14

*Student Development in Nursing Education*                       202

Rules and Regulations                                               205
Students' Rights and Freedoms                                       206
Student Involvement                                                 209
Student Housing                                                     210
Student Activities                                                  212
Student Government                                                  214

Chapter 15

*Student Personnel Services: Program Evaluation*                216

Criteria for Program Evaluation                                     216
Participants in the Evaluation Process                              220
Examples of Evaluation Studies                                      221
General Observations on the Evaluation Process                      226
Bibliography (Part 3)                                               228

Appendix

*Joint Statement On Rights and Freedoms of Students*            234

Preamble                                                            234
I. Freedom of Access to Higher Education                            234
II. In the Classroom                                                235
A. Protection of Freedom of Expression                         235

     B. *Protection Against Improper Academic Evaluation*     235
     C. *Protection Against Improper Disclosure*     235
  III. Student Records     235
  IV. Student Affairs     236
     A. *Freedom of Association*     236
     B. *Freedom of Inquiry and Expression*     236
     C. *Student Participation in Institutional Government*     237
     D. *Student Publications*     237
  V. Off-Campus Freedom of Students     238
     A. *Exercise of Rights of Citizenship*     238
     B. *Institutional Authority and Civil Penalties*     238
  VI. Procedural Standards in Disciplinary Proceedings     238
     A. *Standards of Conduct Expected of Students*     239
     B. *Investigation of Student Conduct*     239
     C. *Status of Student Pending Final Action*     239
     D. *Hearing Committee Procedures*     239

*Index*     241

# Part 1

# *Counseling*

# Chapter 1

# Counseling:
# A Base of Operations

## WHAT IS COUNSELING?

Inevitably, in a book of this sort, one is confronted with the knotty question of trying to define counseling. Indeed, the problem is one not only of definition, but also of clearly delineating differences between counseling and other helping relationships. Perhaps a good place to begin is with the definition developed by the American Personnel and Guidance Association.

> A counseling relationship denotes that the person seeking help retains full freedom of choice and decision, and that the helping person has no authority or responsibility to approve or disapprove of the choices or decisions of the counselee or client.

Another way is to draw a semi-arbitrary line between guidance, counseling, and therapy. Thus we might characterize *guidance* as general in nature, performed individually or in groups—most often the latter—and dealing with information, faculty advising, and group discussions of problem areas. The word "guidance" implies providing external direction for an individual in a decision-making situation rather than assisting him to reach a self-directed decision.

*Counseling* also may involve an individual or a group. It usually deals with the solution of immediate problems, or with the provision of assistance to an individual who requests help in adjusting to some stress situations within his environment. It particularly deals with normative behavior, in that it helps an individual see himself in relation to others. Counseling usually requires a different degree of skill than guidance, for it attempts to deal with feelings and emotions much more than with factual material.

*Therapy* involves the greatest depth and breadth of the three, and also may involve the individual or group. It frequently has as an objective the partial or total reorganization of an individual's personality, and requires the highest skill and degree of training of the three. It particularly deals with pathological behavior in that it is designed to help an individual whose current life style or behavior is in sharp conflict with the mores of the majority of society.

It is important in any human relationship to know the objectives toward which the participants are working, and the needs that are being met in the process. Both the individual and his environment must be considered and understood in any behavior analysis. The personality patterns which a person displays to the outside world are affected by his environment. These patterns tend to be displayed on two levels—cognitive and affective. Thus an individual's personality pattern frequently determines the behaviors which may be of concern to him, to us or to society.

If the student, as well as we as teachers or advisors or counselors, is interested in changing this observed or reported behavior, several possible approaches may be used. Let us, for example, describe a situation in the clinical area that may serve to illustrate these approaches. Suppose we have a demanding patient who constantly insists on having his way and gets angry when his demands are not met immediately. We also have an angry student nurse who seems to be having difficulty in handling the situation. As faculty members, we are interested in affecting the student's attitudes and behavior.

1. We may wish to deal with the cognitive personality. This approach is based on the premise that the student is acting as she does because she doesn't know any better. Therefore we need to teach her the necessary skills and information so that she may change. This is the approach most commonly used by a faculty member. In this approach we may urge the student to concentrate on the patient's behavior. What makes the patient angry? What seem to be his needs? How can the student help meet his needs? What are the characteristics and possible causes of anger and demanding behavior?

2. We may wish to deal with the affective personality. This approach is based on the premise that an individual's behavior has its roots in feelings and emotions. .Therefore we need to explore those feelings with the student, assist her in gaining new insights and self-understanding, and thus help her change her behavior in a desired direction. This approach is oriented more toward counseling or therapy. Through this method we try to help the student deal with her feelings. What makes her angry with the patient? How does she generally handle anger? What might she do to decrease her anger in order to be of more help to the patient?

3. We may wish to deal with both the cognitive and affective aspects of personality. Through this approach we try to combine the elements of teaching and counseling. Thus we might deal with the concepts of anger and demanding behavior. We also attempt to help the student look at the patient's behavior and her own to help her reach a deeper understanding of the behavior being demonstrated by each.

4. We may wish to concentrate on the environment. This approach is based on the premise that the environment determines an individual's behavior. Therefore, if we can somehow change or manipulate the environment, we can produce changed behavior. This change in environment may be total (removal from the situation) or may be nothing more than introducing a new, warm, supporting figure into the environment who does things for instead of to the individual. This is usually classified as supportive counseling. If we use this approach we should

concentrate on questions such as these: Is the clinical area crowded? Is the student assigned to too many patients? Are clinical instructors watching the student too closely and putting her under great pressure? Does the student have an examination that day? In other words, are there things in the life of the student or the patient that could be changed in order to change the dynamics of behavior that are being demonstrated?

To continue the discussion of what is counseling, we have to recognize that the relationship between two people—one a counselor or faculty member and the other a student—is hardly a unique one. There are many ways in which one person may help another. For example, physicians, lawyers, therapists, teachers, pastors, and social workers all participate in forms of helping relationships. As part of this helping relationship, a number of words are used to describe the kind of assistance being provided. There are, however, five principal terms which seem to delineate sharply some of the different forms of a relationship. These are interviewing, advising, supporting, guiding, and counseling.

## Interviewing

Interviewing is the process of gathering information from another person to form the basis for employment, admission, placement, diagnosis, or some other action that affects the other person's life. The interviewer uses all the tools and skills at his command, including verbal and psychological assessment, to make the necessary evaluation of the individual. Although an interview may be requested by an individual, it is normally scheduled by the interviewer, who determines the content, direction, and duration of the interview.

For example: "Miss Johnson, we require an interview of all applicants to our school of nursing in order to help us make the wisest decision for each applicant and for the school. Perhaps a good place to begin would be for you to tell me why you want to enter nursing as a career."

The strength of this approach lies in the speed and efficiency with which a skilled interviewer can gather the necessary information from a student. This greatly facilitates situations in which the interviewer has a number of people to see and limited time available.

The weakness of the approach lies in the fact that the meeting is commonly totally dominated by the interviewer. The student tends to feel threatened or overwhelmed by the obvious control exercised by the interviewer. Interviewing tends to foster feelings of frustration, impotence, and fatalism in a student, for she frequently is never given the opportunity to ask questions or explain herself fully.

## Advising

Advising is the process of assisting another person to deal with a concern, solve a problem or decide upon a course of action. The advisor draws on information and experience available to him to determine the best possible course of action the advisee or student ought to take. The primary source of judgment and evaluation is the advisor. This tends to be one of the most common relationships in an individual's life.

For example: "I see that you had some problems with math in high school. You have voiced concern about having to take statistics next semester. Perhaps it would be helpful for you to take a course in math or algebra this semester." Another example might be: "I understand that you are worried about failing statistics. Your grades so far in the course are very low. You seem to be having a great deal of difficulty and are in danger of failing. You may need to talk with your instructor and arrange for some special tutoring. Another alternative would be to drop the course, take a math course, and then repeat statistics. However, I think it would be best to talk first with your instructor."

The strength of this approach lies in the fact that it is quick. Further, whatever recommendations are made have a high probability of success if the advisor is competent and the advice is taken and followed by the student.

The weakness lies in the fact that the value system of the advisor is dominant. Often the advisee doesn't follow advice. Some advisees become overdependent on the advisor, and fail to develop their ability to be self-directing. This can be a great weakness for someone who hopes to become a competent nurse. When plans fail, it is easy for the advisee to place the blame on the advisor rather than to change plans or alter directions. Advice tends to be the easiest thing in the world to give, and the hardest to accept. If our intent is to produce highly skilled, innovative, self-directing nurses as graduates of our schools, then the process of giving advice would seem to be self-defeating.

## Supporting

Supporting is the process of encouraging another person to continue actions or behave in certain ways. The usual way of providing support is for the person who supports, e.g. instructor, counselor, employer, to express approval or provide rewards when the student behaves in ways which the supporter desires to encourage. The listener may use a nod of the head, expressions of interest, praise or more tangible rewards when the person being supported is behaving or has behaved in ways believed by either person to be inappropriate or self-defeating.

For example: "You did extremely well on your obstetrics exam, and your work in the clinical area has greatly improved in the last two weeks. You are showing better organization and assessment of your patients' needs. I know you have been spending more time with your nursing care plans, and the results are evident in your execution of patient care. I hope you continue to perform at this level. Have you considered the possibility of specializing in maternity nursing?"

The strength of this approach lies in the fact that there is abundant evidence which indicates that this procedure is effective in increasing the supported behavior and suppressing behavior that is not supported. It is extremely useful in helping students who must learn to live in and adjust to a situation that cannot be changed, and also in working with students who doubt their own abilities or selves, or who are afraid to experiment with new behavior.

The weakness lies in the fact that the supporter's value system and judgments may tend to be imposed on the person being supported. The freedom of a student to choose her ways of behavior may be limited. If the instructor or counselor is a highly conforming person, she may foster the same behavior in the student, especially since the instructor frequently serves as a role model for students. It is also easy for the student to shift the responsibility for behavior that has proved to be ineffective. Nevertheless, when used by an experienced faculty member, supporting is a technique that can be quite effective in individual cases.

## Guiding

Guiding is the process of providing another person with the information necessary to deal with concerns, solve a problem or decide on a course of action. The instructor or advisor who provides guidance gives the information that will be helpful to an individual or group making decisions. She decides what information is relevant, and interprets the information to the student who is trying to reach a decision. The information is selected and presented in a form believed to be the most useful for the recipient. This explanation amplifies somewhat our earlier definition of guidance.

For example: "You have indicated an interest in continuing your education after graduation. You will leave here with an Associate in Arts degree. I see from your overall academic record here that you have better than a B average. Your test results indicate that you seem to have the necessary ability to succeed in college. We have here in the office a list of all collegiate programs in nursing. I would recommend that you review the list of schools and see which ones interest you. Also, it would be useful if you talked with faculty members in the department of nursing at the nearby college to get a picture of a typical program, and to become familiar with career opportunities for baccalaureate graduates in nursing. We also have information on various forms of financial assistance available to you. Why don't you review this material, and we can talk further."

The strength of this approach lies in the fact that all decisions are left to the student being guided. She has the benefit of the knowledge, information, and experience of the instructor or advisor. She has the option of utilizing all, part or none of the information presented.

The weakness is less serious than in the approaches previously mentioned. The process of decision making is left to the student, who may not be capable of making an adequate decision. The faculty member provides the data that she perceives as relevant, which may omit other important material, or which may not have meaning for the student. The process deals primarily with facts, and any emotional factors must usually be dealt with entirely by the student who has a decision to make. This last point is perhaps the main limitation in guidance.

## Counseling

Counseling is a relationship between two people in which the principal goal is responsible and effective self-determination by the student. The faculty member participates with the student in resolving a conflict, solving a problem, making a decision or facilitating greater understanding. The relationship is the unique element of counseling. The faculty member believes that the student can and should have primary responsibility for resolving the situation that brings her in to talk with the instructor. The faculty member and the student are co-workers in the process, and each has a stake in the outcome. The student brings in and shares her concern, and the instructor makes an effort to understand the student's point of view, both emotionally and objectively. The faculty member provides information, and interpretations of the information, as it is relevant to the student's concern *from the student's frame of reference.*

Let us turn for an example to our earlier situation of the angry, demanding patient and the angry student. "Miss Johnson, since caring for Mr. Black in 217, you seem to be pretty angry and upset. I can understand how patients can sometimes make me pretty angry. I have found that as I understand my anger better, I am better able to handle it and thus provide better patient care. Do you think we might talk about what made you angry? Perhaps together we can work out some ways of handling situations like this."

The strengths in this approach are several. The value of the assistance given extends beyond the decision of the moment. The student clarifies her own goals and objectives and gains a deeper understanding of herself, her goals, and the relation of her present actions to the future. She learns how to relate information to her concerns, and to make decisions based on the process. She becomes capable of more independent action. Counseling deals primarily with the present and the future. It also deals with both objective facts and emotional aspects as they relate to a student's given situation.

There are also several weaknesses in this approach. Counseling as described up to this point obviously requires more time than any of the other approaches previously mentioned. Counseling gives primary concern to the individual, not to the institution. Therefore the student might well make decisions that are not in the best interest of the institution in choosing actions that may be of the greatest benefit to her. The term "counseling" has also tended to become associated with psychotherapy, and as a consequence may be perceived by the student as something provided only for the weak or the emotionally ill. This connotation makes it difficult to develop the necessary helping relationship with many people.

WHY COUNSEL?

To raise the question as to why counseling services should be provided to our students may seem a little illogical or a non sequitur in a book partially written about counseling. There are schools and colleges which do not believe in providing such services as an integral part of their educational program. They feel that an educational institution should not be in the business of providing therapy. They also feel that if a student's concerns are interfering with her performance, she should obtain help elsewhere or leave the school until she has straightened herself out. On the other hand, there are those who feel that as educators they have a responsibility to do everything possible to facilitate learning, including removal of barriers to learning for their students; that counseling, if indicated or requested, is a legitimate part of the educational process. There is no single correct answer to these questions. Rather, the answer lies in the educational climate and fundamental philosophy of each school, and must evolve from and be continually re-evaluated by the administration, faculty, and students of each school.

We must recognize, in considering such questions, certain well established facts which must be given careful consideration, and which should have a definite impact on the statement of philosophy and ongoing practices within each school.

1. It is not uncommon in many schools of nursing to lose 30 to 40 per cent of the entering freshman class prior to graduation. The staff of the NLN Measurement and Evaluation Service reported in *Nursing Outlook* (1970) that the attrition rate in diploma programs was 33.4 per cent, in baccalaureate nursing programs 45.3 per cent, and in associate degree programs 50.2 per cent.

2. The tremendous shortage of nurses nationally is resulting in marginal patient care in some places, and in an increasing reliance on paraprofessionals to meet nursing needs.

3. Counseling services may help a student be more receptive to learning, more open in sharing her feelings, and better able to understand and communicate with patients for whom she cares.

4. Although there seems to be no single answer to the problem of attrition in schools of nursing, it would seem that a sound program of counseling services accompanied by appropriate curricular changes may have a significant effect on reducing attrition. This area definitely needs specific research, and will be discussed more fully in Chapter 13.

As has been mentioned, the answer to the question of the need for and provision of counseling services requires careful evaluation and research within each school with all who will provide or use such services involved in the evaluation. Some specific techniques for organizing and evaluating a guidance and counseling program will be discussed later. Suffice it to say at this point that all available evidence seems to indicate that, as helping relationships, some form of counseling services seems to have as vital a part to play in the educational growth and development of students as do most of the academic and clinical experience to which a student is exposed.

## WHEN TO COUNSEL

The question about when to provide counseling assistance to a student is frequently raised by nursing educators. Obviously, if a student comes in for assistance, we try to provide it to the best of our ability. But what if the student does not come in? We have all seen students who for one reason or another we felt were in trouble, but who had not asked for help. It is of course always possible that our perception may have been incorrect. It is also possible that we may have been right, but the student was unaware that she had a problem or was not yet ready to seek help in handling it. It is our opinion that forced counseling is not the most effective way to provide assistance. Sensing that a student may need help, calling her in, and saying something such as, "In watching you for the past few days, I have the feeling that something is bothering you. Tell me what it is so I can help," will usually be ineffective. If the student has no problem, she will wonder why you called her in, and sometimes wonder what's the matter with you. Even if you are right, such a statement tends to place a student on the defensive. If she isn't ready for counseling, she will back off and deny that anything is wrong.

There are times, however, when it would seem desirable for a faculty member to call a student in, most often when you, whether as an advisor or an instructor, perceive certain danger signals that may indicate that counseling is needed or may be helpful. These can be described as follows:

1. **Grade Deficiencies.** In order to be admitted to a school of nursing, students must pass certain tests, such as the NLN Pre-Nursing and Guidance Examination, the College Boards or the ACT, which suggest that the applicant is at least average among her peers in terms of tested capacity for learning. Theoretically, this means that given perfect conditions (which seldom prevail), any nursing student has the potential for A or B grades. With this in mind, we must look with suspicion at grades in the D or F level. The same principle holds true in a pass-fail system if the student is failing. When this occurs, several possibilities exist:

   a. The student may be deliberately failing or achieving low grades as a form of punishment or retaliation for parental errors.
   b. The student may not have learned how to study efficiently.
   c. The student may be disinterested in a particular subject.
   d. The student may have been confused at the beginning of a course and never caught up.
   e. The student may be having difficulty adjusting to life away from home.
   f. The student may be having difficulty adjusting to college level teaching processes and pressures.

Regardless of the cause (which may be largely unknown), this may present one kind of situation in which the help of an advisor or instructor is needed. The sort of help given will depend to a large extent on the receptivity of the student and the cause of the specific problem presented.

2. **Inordinate Illness or Absence.**   Illness or class absence may have a variety of causes. In the first place, we should recognize that most student nurses, like most students, have some illness at some time during their program. Further, certain kinds of illness merit close attention. In some cases the illness may be psychosomatic or at least include certain psychological components, e.g. the student who has a pattern of getting sick before or after every examination or testing situation. We must also face the possibility of malingering, and specific fears such as fear of surgery, blood, death. In each instance we must help the student to determine whether she can learn to handle her fears satisfactorily, or whether she cannot anticipate success in the nursing program without extensive therapy which must take place before she continues in the program.

3. **Negative Reports from Peers, Instructors, and Your Own Observations.**   When you or others consistently note that a student shows symptoms of withdrawal behavior, an inability to communicate, or extreme unhappiness or depression, it is probable that she is facing a problem which may benefit from assistance. This does not mean that the prognosis is necessarily good if you take quick action. It is simply a matter of common sense that, as in medicine, assistance provided during the early stages of maladjustment provides greater hope for successful treatment than if secondary symptoms are allowed to develop.

4. **Bizarre Behavior.**   In addition to the foregoing, we must include symptoms of overdependence, the obnoxious personality, drug usage (which we will discuss later in greater detail), stealing, and lying. In each of these situations, counseling would seem to be in order as a first step, supported by referral to a therapist in individual cases.

In the foregoing situations we have talked about the possible need for counseling based on the presenting symptoms. It must be kept in mind, however, that the first contacts may be in another form than counseling, e.g. advising, evaluation conferences, interviewing. Counseling will be initiated only if both the instructor and the student feel that it would be desirable. Even then, the role of the faculty member may still be primarily that of a referral agent.

## BRINGING THE STUDENT IN

What do we do in situations such as the foregoing if the student has not come in for help? The answer to this depends to a large extent on previous relationships between the faculty member and the student. If a relationship has been firmly established, the instructor can be much freer in her approach to the student. We must be careful, however, not to frighten the student off or create problems where none previously existed. Ways of doing this may include the following:

1. "I notice that your grades have been slipping badly lately, and I wanted the chance to talk with you to see if we could perhaps try together to analyze why this is happening. Has something happened that's interfering with your studies, or is there something else affecting your performance that we might be able to do something about?"

2. "When I ran into you earlier this week, I had the feeling that

you were awfully unhappy about something. If my perception is correct, perhaps you'd like to talk about it."

3.   "I understand from several of your classmates who have come to me because of their concern for you that you have been getting pretty upset just before an exam. I'm interested in you and your progress, and thought that perhaps we could talk about how tests make you feel."

In each of these statements the faculty member has called the student in. She is opening the session by indicating the reason for seeing the student, but she is not backing the student into a corner or forcing her to talk. If the student denies that there is a problem, or indicates that she doesn't want any assistance, the instructor may say in the first case, "I'm sorry I misinterpreted what was happening. But since I was concerned, I wanted to try to check it out. If at any time in the future I can be of help, I hope you will let me know." In the second case she may say, "I think I can understand your feelings of not wanting my help at this time. However, I would like to do all I can whenever you are ready. I'll be here, and I hope you'll decide to come back." In both cases the instructor is reinforcing the facts of her caring about the student and her availability. Hopefully, the student will return later when she may feel that the instructor can be of assistance to her.

We must emphasize here that faculty members have, at times, a tendency to read some trauma or psychological problem into every situation. It is well to remember that a wide variation exists in the ability of individuals to act consistently, and that the student nurse who appears to present a problem may very well be acting within what for her is the wide, normal range of reactions. The question to ask yourself is whether the present behavior is unusual for *this* student.

## SUMMARY

In this chapter we have tried to provide an overview of some of the techniques used by faculty members in schools of nursing. With this as a foundation, we can for the moment leave the other forms of helping relationships, and begin to concentrate specifically upon some of the basic elements of counseling.

# Chapter 2

# *Counseling and the Helping Relationship*

In Chapter 1 we discussed counseling and some of the ways it differs from other kinds of helping relationships, such as advising and guiding. It would seem useful at this point to begin to look more closely at counseling. Such an examination should include some of the basic principles of counseling, the ethical standards that cover the counseling relationship, and a beginning look at the instructor-counselor-advisor role. These things, in general, comprise the substance of this chapter.

## PRINCIPLES OF COUNSELING

By principles of counseling, we are really talking about some basic beliefs and practices that form the cornerstone of every counselor's work. These points are important enough to state clearly and explain fully as a foundation for later material. The faculty member who can accept and incorporate into her value system each of these points is well on the road towards effective helping relationships with her students.

1. *There is no single right way to counsel.* There are many counseling philosophies and methods that are equally effective, depending on the two personalities present in each counseling session. For each counseling relationship is a new and unique meeting of two unique personalities—the human interaction between the instructor and the student. Every time a new student comes in, the relationship is different because of the different elements present. Although there are many errors which interfere with effective assistance for a student, there is no single right way. In some respects, effective counseling depends on the approaches which the faculty member finds most comfortable and successful. If these approaches do not work in a given situation or with a given student, then the faculty member can refer to someone else. It must be remembered that the instructor can never be all things to all students.

2. *Student nurses have inner resources to help themselves.* As faculty members, we must believe that each student has the innate capacity to help herself, i.e. the power of self-determination. This does not mean that we don't provide all the assistance we can to students. It does mean that we usually are dealing with "normal" people who may be reacting

quite normally to an abnormal situation in their lives. The instructor may provide the information, the vehicle or the catalyst, but each student has the capacity to solve her own problems or to make the best decisions for herself at the moment.

3. *Start where the student is and accept her as she is.* It is a waste of time to attempt to assist a student by beginning where you think she should be. By starting where she is, you and she can progress together at the same pace. At the same time it is equally important to accept the student as she is rather than try to remake her into your image. Without trying, we exercise a great deal of influence on our students and their lives. We do this by what we say and do. We must be on constant guard that we don't reject a student because her way of life or standards may be or may seem to be very different from ours.

4. *Each student nurse should be respected and her potentialities for growth recognized.* This is a quality that we cannot teach to another human being. It represents a deep basic belief in humanity that is either present or absent. Without it, at best an instructor or a student nurse will be limited to superficial or controlling relationships. With it, there is no limit to the depth, the intensity, the power of the relationship that can develop between the instructor and the student.

5. *The role of the faculty member is not to moralize, to preach, to attempt to impose her own values or the values of the institution or society upon the students.* This does not, of course, mean that the instructor lacks values, but rather that she has the obligation of *not* imposing these values on others. This is what makes counseling different from many other helping relationships. The basic concept of "right" and "wrong" is appropriate only in individual terms. What is right for one person may not be right for another. We have the responsibility of respecting our students' right to believe and act the way they wish as they have the responsibility of respecting our value system. Essentially, the student has the freedom to do anything she wishes with her life as long as it does not infringe upon the rights of others, and as long as she is willing to accept the responsibility for and consequences of her actions. The instructor's role may be to provide information and alternatives so that the student may make the best decision for her, but the final decision always rests with the student.

Peer "right" vs. individual "right" has long presented problems for students; the same is true in the area of perceptions. For example, a student nurse came in and said, "I think that I am immature." When the instructor asked her why she was concerned, and if she really believed that she was in fact immature, the student said, "No, but several of my instructors told me that I am." As she continued to work with the instructor, she began to see that her own beliefs were all that mattered, and that it might be more profitable to explore what in her behavior may have caused the instructors to arrive at an incorrect judgment.

A male student came in wondering whether there was something wrong with him. He had refused to go to bed with a girl he was dating, and she had told him there must be something wrong with him. He felt that she was drunk, and although he enjoyed sex, he could not see taking advantage of a situation in which the girl had to get drunk so that she could do something she would have felt too guilty about if sober.

Women students frequently express deep concerns about conflicts between personal standards and peer standards. They say, "I talked with some of the other girls in my class, and they say I am old-fashioned, that there is nothing wrong with premarital sex. I was raised differently, and I think it is wrong. But now I don't know, I'm not sure."

From a moral or legal point of view the student's behavior may be wrong, but not from a counseling point of view. If this is her decision, rationally arrived at, of how she wishes to lead her life, this is her right regardless of how society may view her actions. This is frequently a difficult concept for a novice in counseling to understand and accept. It is almost a cardinal rule of counseling, however, and is a vital part of successful counseling. Essentially, we are trying to foster the development of the inner-directed person of David Riesman or the self-actualizing person of Abraham Maslow. The student has many other people in her life whose primary role is to teach her, correct her, advise her, punish her or judge her. Hopefully, the instructor who is doing counseling will be unique in that she does none of these at this time with this student.

6. *The faculty member providing counseling should listen with an emphasis on nonevaluation.* This refers to the ability to listen with an open mind rather than a closed mind to what the student is really saying. Why is she telling me this? What does she seem to be feeling? What is she really asking? There are many times when you may be unable to answer these questions, but it is important to try. Probably the greatest weakness of beginning counselors is their concentration on factual statements of the counselee rather than the underlying feelings being expressed verbally and nonverbally. This is the same principle that applies in nurse-patient relationships that we try to teach to students. As instructors know, it is much easier to teach students to respond to the content expressed by a patient than it is to develop the sensitivity to identify and respond to feelings. As faculty members, we sometimes have the same difficulty in our relationships with students.

## ETHICAL STANDARDS OF COUNSELING

In discussing the Ethical Standards of the Counselor, as prepared by the American Personnel and Guidance Association (1961), we do so knowing that most nursing educators who read this book will not be full-time counselors. Yet it is our firm belief that these standards apply equally well when adapted to cover nursing educators who provide counseling services, whether on a full-time or part-time basis. Only if these standards are followed is there a climate for the counseling relationship to develop to its fullest potential.

1. The faculty member's *primary* obligation when counseling is to respect the integrity and promote the welfare of the student with whom she is working.

In other words, everything we do through counseling is for the student's welfare, and nothing we do should ever be used against her or to hurt her. We are working with her to the best of our ability. We must remember at this point that we are human, we are fallible. The counseling relationship is a two-way sharing process. Both participants may have similar problems, needs, beliefs, feelings, and so forth, but one is able to set her own concerns aside to help the other. The faculty member doing counseling is not a small god sitting on high and dispensing panaceas and magic solutions from the depths of her wisdom. Instead, both members of a counseling relationship give to and receive from each other with as much mutual trust and openness as can grow between two people.

2. The counseling relationship and information resulting therefrom must be kept confidential consistent with the obligations undertaken by the faculty member as a professional person.

The important word here is "confidential." The information you may receive from a student through counseling is confidential, will not be released, and will never be used to hurt her. This understanding of the meaning of confidentiality ideally would be understood and supported by faculty and administration, and would be conveyed during an orientation to counseling given to all students. Otherwise, it is clearly agreed to with the individual student at the very outset of the relationship. This also means that the instructor is not free to discuss a student's concerns indiscriminately, e.g. in the faculty lounge. There are provisions for professional consultation, and a safety clause that we will discuss a little later.

3. Records of the counseling relationship, including interview notes, test data, correspondence, tape recordings, and other documents, are to be considered professional information for use in counseling, research, or the teaching of faculty members doing counseling, but always with the full protection of the identity of the student, and with precaution so that no harm will come to her.

This covers the same safeguards that apply to the use of patient data. If, for example, you are conducting an in-service training program in your school to help faculty members develop better counseling skills, you must be careful about using material from actual students within your own school. The only way you can do this ethically would be if you can completely protect the identity of the student. You should also secure the permission of the student in writing in advance of any such use in or out of the school. One important point that should be stressed here is that counselors in general have no legal immunity in most states to enable them to maintain confidences. All records and other material can be subpoenaed by court order. This means that faculty members doing counseling must be extremely careful as to what records they maintain on students, and who is given access to them.

4. The student should be informed of the conditions under which she may receive counseling assistance at or before the time she enters the counseling relationship. This is particularly true in the event of conditions which the student would not likely be aware of.

In other words, when a student comes in and asks you if she can talk with you, she is in effect saying, "I would like to be able to talk with you in confidence, to bring things out in the open, and say things secure in the knowledge that you won't repeat them to others." If there are any institutional or other restrictions on your ability to maintain such a confidence, you have the obligation of informing the student of this immediately.

5.   As with medical consultation, the faculty member doing counseling reserves the right to consult with any other professionally competent person about a student.

If a student wishes to talk with you, both you and she always have the right to consult with someone else if either of you feels in a particular situation that she is uncomfortable or needs additional assistance. Such consultation is always sought solely for the benefit of the student. If a faculty member uses a colleague or someone else in the same institution as a consultant, great care should be taken to maintain anonymity of the student if possible, and to reveal only what is necessary to obtain proper consultative help. Special precaution should be taken not to use someone as a consultant who currently has or who will have in the future a relationship with the student in a teaching, administrative or clinical role. This potentially may place the student in jeopardy, depending on the consultant's use of the information.

6.   The faculty member shall decline to initiate or shall terminate a counseling relationship when she cannot be of professional assistance to the student because of lack of competence, severity of the problem, or feelings of personal limitations. In such instances the faculty member shall refer the student to someone else qualified to provide the needed assistance. In the event the student declines the suggested referral, the faculty member is not obligated to continue the counseling relationship.

If you feel that you are not competent to assist a student when she comes to see you, then you have an obligation to refer her to someone else. If the student presents one problem that gradually evolves into areas beyond your ability to help, you have the same obligation to refer. If the student refuses to see someone else, you are ethically under no obligation to continue the relationship. This last situation leads to another point worth mentioning here.

It is recognized that if a student refuses a referral, you can ethically still terminate the counseling relationship. At this point you have to reach the decision as to whether no help (refusal to see someone else) is better or worse than the assistance you can provide within your limited ability. If you feel in such a situation that it is more desirable to continue seeing the student—with the primary objective of bringing her to the point of accepting a referral—then you should definitely plan on professional consultation or supervision for your work with her.

7. When the faculty member learns through counseling relationships of conditions which are likely to harm others over whom her institution has responsibility, she is expected to report *the condition* to the appropriate responsible authority, but in such a manner as not to reveal the identity of her counselee.

This standard is designed to deal with instances in which the situation rather than the individual may be harmful to the institution, e.g. drugs, homosexuality. Basically, this recognizes your dual responsibility to those with whom and for whom you work—your students and your employers. It must be recognized that just as we protect individual rights, so we have an obligation to safeguard the rights of society. This is based on the assumption that the faculty member also has rights, i.e. the right and the authority to decide when to report and what to report. It should be clearly understood by anyone doing counseling what conditions the institution demands be reported. Such things then become limitations that must be communicated to students.

8. In the event that the student's condition is such as to require others to assume responsibility for her, or when there is clear and imminent danger to the student or to others, the faculty member is expected to report this fact to an appropriate responsible authority, or take such other emergency measures as the situation demands.

This represents the only legitimate escape clause that a faculty' member has for legitimately breaking a confidence. You as the counselor are the only one who can interpret what "clear and imminent danger" means to you, and when it applies in a given situation. Although you may have time to consult with someone else, often you have to make an immediate judgment as to what you will do. Even with consultation, you are the only one who can and should make such a judgment, for you are part of the counseling relationship and know the student. What decision you make will usually be a function of your own philosophy, your professional judgment, your personal sense of security, and your biases. It must be understood that no one expects you to be without biases, but justifiably you are expected to be aware of them, to recognize situations in which they may interfere with your judgment and ability to help a student, and to refer or seek help whenever appropriate. It is vitally important if you decide to break confidentiality that you tell the student that you must do so and why you must do so. If possible, the student should be given the option of reporting the information herself rather than having you do it. If you are unable to consult with the student prior to revealing the information, it is important to see the student as soon as possible to tell her that the information was revealed. Breaking confidence is never an easy decision to make, and it should be given careful thought before it is done.

## CHARACTERISTICS OF THE COUNSELOR

Carl Rogers, one of the leading psychotherapists in the country for the past 20 years, has written extensively about the counseling relationship. He has, among other things, been particularly interested in the characteristics of both the counselor and the counseling relationship that contribute to or inhibit the development of a sound helping relationship. He raises certain questions that anyone who does counseling—or for that matter, anyone working in any form of helping relationship—must ask herself and answer honestly. These were expressed initially in his book *On Becoming a Person* (1961), and can be applied to the instructor-student, counselor-counselee, nurse-patient or any other form of human interaction.

1. Can I function in a manner which will be perceived by the other person as trustworthy, as dependable, as a caring fellow human being? Is this the way I can actually be in everything I do so that she can legitimately and rightfully depend on me as a professional person?

2. Can I be expressive enough as a person so that what I am will be communicated unambiguously, so that I am verbally and physically everything I say and do in a helping relationship, so that what I am and all that I am will be communicated to the student (or patient) clearly and honestly?

3. Can I let myself experience positive attitudes toward this other person—attitudes of warmth, caring, liking, interest, respect, love? Can I, in general, let myself experience positive attitudes toward others around me? We ask our patients, our students, and our counselees to respect us, to trust us, to believe in us, but this needs to be mutual. We equally have to be able to respect them, trust them, and believe in them as individuals, genuinely and sincerely. We may not approve of everything a student does, but we can, nevertheless, still like her as an individual. We ask each student with whom we work when she comes to us to let down the walls behind which she lives, to let herself become free enough to share with us her genuine feelings, emotions, and fears. But can we rightfully ask this of a student if we are not equally ready and able to do the same with her, and allow her to see us as a person rather than as a cold, authoritarian individual? We know that it is not uncommon for a student to develop strong positive feelings toward a faculty member. But if we can overcome our fear of experiencing similar positive feelings reciprocally, then it is entirely possible in certain situations for us to be definitely attracted to the student or patient. There is nothing inherently wrong in this. Rather, it means that we are not afraid of our own feelings, as we are not afraid of the feelings a student or patient may express to us.

4. Can I be strong enough as a person to be separate from those with whom I work? Am I secure enough within myself to permit them their separateness? Am I strong enough to remain sufficiently apart from the student or patient to maintain my objectivity, and at the same time be secure enough within myself not only to permit but also to encourage her separateness and independence? Whether in a teaching or counseling relationship, we are not trying to foster feelings of dependency. Rather, we learn to exercise control so that we do not become emotionally involved with a student or patient to the extent that our judgment becomes faulty. We are not afraid to get off the shore and into the same boat with the student, but if the boat begins to sink, we don't go down with it. Unless our judgment can remain sound and objective, we become of little help to the student or patient, and, in many cases, to ourselves. If we find that our judgment begins to be clouded, we must be wise, sensitive, and free enough to refer the student to someone else who may be better able in the given situation to be objective and helpful.

5. Can I let myself enter fully into the world of her feelings and

personal meanings and see these as she does? Can I openly and freely and fully enter into her world instead of demanding that she enter mine? Can I accept each facet of this other person which she presents to me, or do I in effect say, "I can accept this but not that"? Acceptance does not mean that I necessarily condone or approve of a particular action. Rather, it means that I continue to accept nonjudgmentally the total person with whom I am working. Unfortunately, for most of us there aren't very many people around who will really listen to us in a nonjudgmental fashion. Can we provide this to the student or patient with whom we are working?

6. Can I act with sufficient sensitivity in the relationship that my behavior will not be perceived as a threat? It is easy for a student to be threatened and fearful of what we say, by what we do or by who we are. Can I try to minimize or free her from the threat of external evaluation? Can I make her see that, in the counseling relationship, I am not here to judge her, to evaluate her, but rather to work with her and her ability to work through her concerns of the moment? Can I accept this other individual as a person who is in the process of becoming, or will I be shackled by her past and by my past? I must, as a counselor and as a faculty member, be able to recognize this other individual as a fellow human being who is constantly striving for something worthwhile in her life. She changes and adapts to meet the situations, the demands, the stresses in her life. We both may have similar needs, concerns, and fears. We both have within us the capacity for growth and change. Therefore neither of us has the right to judge the other by our or her past, only to help the other fulfill the promise of the future.

## THE CORE OF THE HELPING RELATIONSHIP

Giffen (1969) stresses the importance of the concept of trust in an effective interpersonal relationship, and describes the potential interference with or barrier to communication of a neutral professional manner, an attitude of superiority or of dogmatic certainty. Giffen believes that the counselor must have above-average amounts of empathy, warmth, and genuineness. Giffen's point ties in nicely with our discussion of Rogers' characteristics of the counselor.

Rogers has been identified as the founder of a particular school or philosophy of counseling. It is not our intention here or elsewhere to discuss counseling theories or philosophies, for that is another book. Nor is it our intention to ask our readers to adopt the philosophy or ideas of Carl Rogers. We have chosen the points previously covered in this chapter because they apply equally well not only to all counselors regardless of their orientation, but also in many ways to any human relationship that operates on a deep, sensitive, empathic level. Rogers has looked at not only his own beliefs, but also those of other counselors who operate from a different frame of reference than his. In so doing, he freely admits that other approaches to counseling may be equally effective. He identified what he believed to be the common elements in all counseling approaches regardless of the orientation of the counselor.

These commonalities he attempted to reduce into five key points which he defines as the core elements of any helping relationship. In many ways these five points serve to synthesize much of the previous discussion.

The first of these elements is called *congruence*. This he defined as "that the counselor is what he is; in the relationship with the counselee he is genuine and without front or facade, openly being the feelings and attitudes which at the moment are flowing in him." The counselor is what he is, rather than what he thinks he should be or what he thinks someone else wants him to be. This means that the counselor is aware of what and who he is, is aware of his strengths and weaknesses, his biases, and his set of values. He is genuine and consistent in his relationships with other people, whether they be counselees, family, friends, colleagues or casual acquaintances. True congruence means that the counselor is able to be what and who he is in all human relationships, not just his professional ones.

The second element is identified as *empathy*. This is defined as "the counselor experiences an accurate empathic understanding of his counselee's private world, and is able to communicate some of the significant fragments of that understanding." The counselor in essence is saying, "I can honestly say that I can understand how you feel, and I think that I can feel this with you." This is not sympathy which tends to become subjective, for, unlike sympathy, our own emotions do not get in the way. This is understanding—an accurate perception of the private world of another human being. "Even though I am not living in your world with you, even though I am external to it, even though I cannot say I know exactly how you feel and share the same feelings with you, nevertheless I think I can understand how you feel."

The third element is identified as *positive regard*. This is based on the belief that growth and change are more likely to occur the more the counselor experiences and communicates a warm, positive, acceptant attitude toward what lies within the counselee. He prizes the counselee as a unique, feeling individual. "I value this individual who is working here with me. I do not feel that she or her problems are beneath me or unworthy of my attention. I do not feel that she is a waste of my time. She is valuable, and if I can be of any help to her, then I have fulfilled my role. While I am with her, she is the most important person in the world to me."

The fourth element, an extension of the third, is *unconditionality of regard*. The more the positive regard described above is unconditional, the greater the effectiveness of the relationship. The counselor does not accept certain feelings or actions and disapprove of others; his acceptance is unconditional. "I accept everything about the counselee, not just part of her and her feelings. If I cannot accept her unconditionally because of my filters, my biases, then I must help her find another who may be more able than I to provide her with this openness and unconditionality."

The final and most crucial element is the *counselee's perception*. Unless these common elements and attitudes have been in some degree communicated to the counselee, and perceived by her, they do not exist for her and thus cannot be effective. For example, a faculty member in a school of nursing who functions as a teacher, a faculty advisor, and a part-time counselor or administrator may feel that she can separate these roles, and she may actually be able to do so successfully. Nevertheless if this separation cannot be perceived and experienced by the student, then it doesn't exist for her; as far as she is concerned, there is no separation. If you see yourself as a warm, accepting, understanding person, and the student does not, this doesn't necessarily mean that you are wrong. It may mean that the way you are may not be communicated successfully to the student because of your methods of communicating, her methods of receiving, or a combination of both. Constructive change and growth seem to occur only when the student perceives and experiences a certain psychological climate in the relationship. The conditions which produce this climate do not consist of knowledge, intellectual training, orientation in some phiolsophy of counseling, or technique. Rather, they represent feelings and attitudes which must be deeply and genuinely experienced by the counselor, and perceived by the student, if they are to be effective in fostering a helping relationship.

## THE COUNSELOR, THE TEACHER, AND THE NURSE

The majority of the readers of this book serve all three roles described in the title of this section—they are occasionally counselors to their students or patients; they are teachers sharing knowledge and skills with students and patients; and they are or have been nurses ministering to the needs of patients. In addition, they may fill a variety of other roles in their life as women, wives, mothers, friends, and so on. In each of the roles mentioned, the reader is actively involved in a human relationship with others; in many instances this takes the form of a helping relationship. Even though every situation and relationship tends somewhat to be unique, there are some common elements in the three principal roles. Describing these may help to eliminate some of the role confusion that inevitably faces the beginner in the counseling field. It may also help by indicating some of the ways in which the counselor may be a unique person in the life of an individual.

1. The counselor does her best to avoid judgments and evaluations of the student. The teacher must, by the necessity of her role, evaluate the student's progress and knowledge. The nurse must continually evaluate the physical condition of her patient to determine significant change or progress.

2. The counselor will share all the information she possesses with the student to help the student move toward greater self-understanding or decision making. The teacher will share all information with a student that she feels the student needs to know. The nurse frequently will withhold information from a patient upon the judgment of the health team.

3. The counselor tries always to start at the level of the student, and move with her at the student's pace. The teacher usually starts where the student is, but pushes the student to progress at the rate determined

by the teacher. The nurse always starts where the patient is, and tries to encourage the patient to move toward self-care as soon as possible.

4. The counselor has as her primary obligation the welfare of the student. The teacher may at times have to subordinate the welfare of an individual student to the welfare of the group. The nurse normally has as her primary obligation the welfare of the patient, but this is determined by her and the other members of the health team.

5. The counselor may use measurement and evaluation tools in consultation with the student for diagnosis, self-understanding, or to provide more information to the student. The teacher uses measurement and evaluation tools at her discretion, normally without consulting with the student. The nurse, either alone or on instructions from a physician, will frequently use diagnostic tools to help determine the course of treatment. Ideally, the patient is consulted and given a thorough rationale for the tests given.

6. The counselor normally works on a one-to-one basis, but may on occasion become involved in group work. The teacher normally works on a group basis, but may on occasion work on a tutorial one-to-one basis. The nurse almost always works on a one-to-one basis, although she is usually responsible for a group at the same time.

7. The counselor's contacts with a student are usually private and invariably confidential. The teacher's contacts with a student are usually in a classroom or clinical situation, and information gathered is usually used as a part of the broad evaluation process. The nurse's contacts with a patient may be private or in a ward situation, and information gathered is usually shared with the other members of the health team and entered in the medical history.

8. The counselor keeps records that are confidential, are generally unavailable to others, and are used solely to assist the student. The teacher keeps records that are available to other faculty members and administrators who desire information about a student. The nurse maintains records that are always accessible to other members of the health disciplines working with the same patient.

9. The counselor usually sees a counselee at the student's request or initiation. The teacher sees a student when either she or the student feels the need. The nurse usually sees a patient on a regularly scheduled basis regardless of the wishes of the patient.

10. The counselor tries to understand and work with the whole individual within her environment. The teacher is primarily concerned with the student's level of knowledge and performance. The nurse is primarily concerned with the patient's physical condition, although as part of total patient care she will be equally concerned with other needs of the patient.

## COUNSELING: WHO DOES IT?

We have been talking a great deal up to this point about counseling and the counselor, but we really have not identified who actually does the counseling in schools of nursing. This does not mean to imply that there is only one pattern, but rather that in many instances a combination of patterns may best meet the needs within a particular school of nursing. We also have to recognize that there may be different forms of counseling assistance available to students just as there are different kinds of counseling—educational-vocational and personal-social—although many times the types and forms of problems become so interrelated that they cannot be categorized.

Educational counseling is tied in very much with academic advising. In most institutions we find faculty members and advisors handling educational and vocational guidance, and academic advising. In most cases, however, such persons are not equipped to provide personal-social counseling. On the next level may be the part-time or full-time counselor. This may be a faculty advisor selected for this role because of personality, interest, and training, or someone recruited from outside the school of nursing. On the advanced level we have the highly trained resource personnel who are available for referrals from the school. Let us look at the most common sources of assistance available to students by progressing from the unskilled to the highly skilled.

1. **The Family and Society.** Frequently students in trouble will seek help from within their family, their church or perhaps their family physician. This is usually because the student does not feel free enough to go to anyone within the school or college. It will also frequently occur among first-year students who have not yet really severed the strong dependency ties on home, family, and community. Assistance obtained from these sources may be quite satisfactory, depending on the nature of the problem, although most such sources are persons who operate out of minimal or no professional training in counseling (this is changing rapidly among students presently enrolled in seminaries and medical schools), and most importantly tend to operate out of a closed-value system. Students most commonly will get a great deal of advice, some information and guidance, and little professional, confidential, nonjudgmental counseling from such sources.

2. **The Peer Group.** Starting in high school, the peer group begins to assume a role of overwhelming importance and influence in the life of a student. She tends to turn to friends within the group for opinions, advice, a good listener, and so forth. This can be an excellent source of support or a prime source of rejection for individual students. Obviously, help from this source is usually highly subjective, and highly loaded with value statements such as, "I think you should," "I would if I were you," "Why don't you because everyone else is," and the like. Students can be helped to become more effective supports for each other by building on the communication skills which are a part of every nurse's education. The same skills we encourage her to use with patients can be used in a helpful manner with fellow students—skills such as the ability to listen, to avoid preaching, to know when to refer to someone more competent than she. Since this source of help for students will always be a factor, it makes sense to try to introduce some basic counseling skills into the communications sequence.

Unfortunately, this is an area that is not particularly strong in many schools. Graduates of our schools of nursing today are expected to be highly skilled professionals able to provide total care for their patients. But if we look at the educational patterns in many schools of nursing, we find students taking a general course in psychology, a general course in sociology, and perhaps one or two electives in the behavioral sciences. Therefore the hope has to lie in what is taught under the broad heading of communications skills. This is one of the less effective parts of nursing education, owing to the failure in many schools to utilize the resources available to them in other departments of the college or university, or within the community. You are well aware as you read this book of your own limitations in preparation to counsel your students. As you look at your curriculum, is there any more being done today than in your own education to prepare students better? Better preparation could not only increase the effectiveness of the nurse-patient relationship, but would also greatly assist faculty members and advisors of the future to do a more effective job of working with students.

3. **The Faculty Member.** Regardless of the availability of other sources of help, students will inevitably seek out individual faculty members. Burton (1962) found that counseling in many schools of nursing is part of the function of instructors, many of whom feel inadequately prepared for this responsibility. She recognizes that counseling students will require the expenditure of additional time and effort by faculty members; however, the improved emotional adjustment of students may result in a lowered attrition rate and more effective nursing service. Killen and Nehren (1967) feel that any instructor is qualified to counsel if she is interested in people, if she listens, if she is emotionally supportive, and skillful in problem-solving techniques. They recognize that instructors vary in their abilities, and will not always be consistent in different situations and with different people. They found students particularly coming to faculty members with concerns in the areas of education, finances, interpersonal relationships, intrapersonal relationships, and religion. They conclude that the counselor must understand her own feelings, and how she feels about concepts such as dependency, authority, anger, guilt, and anxiety.

We are not referring here to the assigned faculty advisor. We have already mentioned that counseling ideally should be on a voluntary basis rather than be compulsory, because in assigning students to an advisor you may run into personality clashes, or a student may feel more at ease talking with a faculty member other than her assigned advisor. The student may have you, her faculty advisor, in a particular sequence, and not want to risk coming to you to talk about her concerns reflecting on her professional competence. Nevertheless giving each student the freedom to seek out any faculty member may create some problems. Inevitably, students tend to gravitate toward certain faculty members who have great facility in establishing close, helping relationships. As a result, such faculty members tend to be overloaded since they must maintain their instructional responsibilities as well. It should be emphasized that even though a faculty member may be involved in only occasional counseling, during such times she is bound by the same ethical standards that apply to the full-time counselor. If you find certain faculty members who are natural resources for students by virtue of their interest, skill, and personality, then it would be desirable to try to provide them with released time to do counseling, while encouraging them to seek advanced training in counseling.

4. **The Faculty Advisor.**   Assignment of an advisor is one of the most common practices in most schools and colleges. We have already mentioned the problem of assigned faculty advisors and personality clashes. The practice of dividing the student body up and assigning a certain number of advisees equally among the faculty is being criticized more and more today. The problem is not a new one. A number of years ago Feder (1949) wrote:

> To be realistic we must recognize that many teachers are basically neither interested nor skilled in dealing with individual students and their problems. Furthermore, some faculty members . . . should not, because of their own personality organization or disorganization, be allowed to engage in the deep personal contacts characteristic of the counseling situation.
>
> It is necessary to make a clear-cut distinction between the faculty advisor whose function is chiefly assisting with registration procedures, and the faculty counselor who, by virtue of special training, interest, and assignment, spends an allotted portion of his time dealing with student adjustment.

Another problem mentioned earlier in this chapter is the perception of the student. Even though a faculty advisor may feel that she can separate her advising, teaching, and counseling roles, if the student does not perceive and accept this separation, then it does not exist in practice and will hinder if not stop any development of a counseling relationship. It should also be mentioned here that, as with faculty members, faculty advisors are also bound by the same ethical standards for counselors whenever they agree to enter a counseling relationship with a student.

5. **The Part-Time Counselor.**   Here we are talking about two different models. The first is the faculty member with released time to do part-time counseling. We have already discussed some of the inherent weaknesses in this plan. The second is represented by an individual who comes to the school of nursing on a part-time basis, i.e. one or two days a week, to provide counseling services. Ideally, it would be better to have either a full-time visiting counselor or a dual teacher-counselor than just a part-time visiting counselor, for several reasons. First, when a student feels that she needs help and has finally worked up enough nerve to ask for help, she wants it immediately if at all possible, rather than the following week when the part-time counselor arrives. To students in time of crisis, the availability of immediate assistance is an extremely important factor. Second, each school of nursing can use a full-time person who is intimately aware of all aspects of and personalities within the school. Such awareness is almost impossible for a part-time person to achieve. It should be pointed out here that a highly skilled part-time counselor can be a valuable adjunct as a referral agent for counseling

services provided within the school of nursing. If used as a part of a comprehensive counseling program, the part-time counselor can be quite effective.

6. **The Full-Time Counselor.**   This would seem to be the most desirable pattern for nursing education. There is no evidence to support the idea that such an individual be a nurse. A full-time counselor avoids any of the problems of role conflict and lack of professional training described earlier. The counselor is not a clinical psychologist, but she has training and skills which equip her to handle the normal patterns and concerns of a basically normal student population. She relies heavily on the information she receives from faculty members, and serves as a resource and referral agent for those faculty members seeing students for short-term advising and counseling. She in turn may be supported by a wide variety of referral agents to whom she can turn for additional help. In essence, the full-time counselor represents the second line of defense for students in need of help who are unable, for a variety of reasons, to obtain such help from sources previously mentioned in this section.

7. **Referral Resources.**   At least some of these are always available to any student, faculty member or counselor who needs additional assistance. They include a wide range of services, some of which are undoubtedly available in any community that has a school of nursing. Such resources may include the following types of services:

College counseling center
College health center
Community mental health center
Family service agencies
Private psychologists and psychiatrists
Hospital psychiatric staff
College psychology or counseling departments
School counselors and school psychologists
Private physicians
Clergy and college chaplains
Drug treatment centers
Other counselors

Such a list is not necessarily all-inclusive. One of the responsibilities of a full-time counselor or a school of nursing guidance committee is to compile and keep up to date a readily available list of referral resources available within the school, college or surrounding community at large. How and when to utilize such resources effectively will be discussed in detail in Chapter 7.

At this point the reader may ask, "But what about me? I am a faculty member who is called upon to do some counseling, and you have just finished showing all the problems inherent in such a role. I was aware of some of them before. But the fact remains that our school does not have a full-time counselor, and has little prospect of one in the foreseeable future.

Even if we are fortunate enough to get one, I undoubtedly will continue to do some counseling."

This is an important question. Obviously, we cannot professionally prepare a counselor by asking someone to read a book. We can, however, do several things. First, we can try to develop to a higher degree the beginning counseling skills and referral skills for those individual faculty members who are doing some counseling. We can do this by covering the basic techniques and principles of counseling, and suggest ways of continued staff development.

Second, we can help such persons become aware of some of the obvious limitations of their role, and develop ways of minimizing the resulting negative effects of such limitations. Third, we can try to help faculty members become more effective *as faculty members* in their contacts with students, and increase their ability to develop an exciting, open educational climate within each school of nursing. At this point it is time to begin to look more closely at the counseling process.

# Chapter 3

# The Counseling Session

In discussing the counseling relationship we are primarily concerned at this point with one-to-one or individual counseling. The counseling session represents the setting in which the counselor and the student come together. From the very first contact between the faculty member and the student, the embryonic relationship may take many forms. It is useful for anyone doing counseling to review the principal stages of a counseling session in order to gain a deeper understanding of some of the techniques that will enhance the development of a helping relationship. Thus the purpose of this chapter is to explore how counseling begins, and to analyze the developmental stages of a counseling session.

## HOW COUNSELING BEGINS

The first necessary step in most counseling relationships is an awareness of the problem or concern on the part of the student. There are many times when we as faculty members may feel that a student has a problem that is affecting her performance, and that she needs help of some sort, but this is only our perception, which may or may not be accurate. The student may not share the same awareness. We are primarily talking here about *readiness for counseling*. The situation may be such that (a) we feel that the student has a problem, but she doesn't recognize it or feel it—in such a case she is not ready for counseling; or (b) the student may indeed recognize that she has a problem, but is not yet ready or does not feel that she can discuss her concern with anyone else.

As faculty members we can call the student in if her performance in class or in the clinical area has slipped. We can teach her and advise her; we can attempt to explore the causes of her changed performance or attitude; we can offer to assist her if something is bothering her, or suggest that she may wish to talk with someone else. Nevertheless, unless the student has reached the point of readiness in such circumstances, we must wait until the student recognizes that she has a problem, has exhausted all her own resources in trying to help herself, and now needs and comes for assistance to the faculty member or counselor. It is admittedly frustrating to a faculty member who sees a student in trouble, but finds that the student refuses all attempts at help or finds the student denying that there is a problem. We have to recognize that many people feel that it is a sign of weakness to seek help—"There is obviously something wrong with me if I need help from someone else; they will think I am really crazy." This is an unfortunate connotation that nevertheless represents a factor we must face. If the fear of going to someone else for assistance is great, then the student will normally wait until the pressure builds to the point where the need for help outweighs all other considerations.

It should be quite obvious that we believe that forced counseling should be avoided when possible. It has been our experience that students assigned to forced counseling for a variety of reasons have great difficulty overcoming the initial barriers to a meaningful relationship. As advisors and instructors we can force students to come in to see us, but we cannot force them to express their feelings and concerns to us. Although it is usually difficult to overcome the initial barriers to communication, forced counseling can at times be effective. In order to do this, the faculty member or counselor should try to do several things. First, the pressure to come in ideally comes from someone other than the counselor. Second, the counselor makes it clear that (a) she has a feeling—*which may be incorrect*–that the student could use some assistance, and (b) that since she is concerned about the student, she would like to help. Remember that we are talking here about counseling. We recognize that there are many occasions in nursing education, particularly in the clinical areas, when an instructor must call a student in. What most commonly occurs in such situations, at least initially, is teaching, advising, guiding or, in extreme cases, discipline. The point that we are trying to make here is that the most effective counseling is usually done when it is requested or initiated by the student. This is the best signal we have of readiness for counseling.

A second stage is to establish a beneficial counseling relationship which makes it possible to really work on a student's problem. A word that is frequently used to describe this stage is *rapport,* i.e. establishing a climate that is right for and conducive to counseling. This includes a physical setting that enhances privacy and confidentiality. The middle of a ward or corridor is hardly the place to instill much confidence or sense of privacy. Establishing this emotional climate takes time. This doesn't mean, however, that the faculty member needs unlimited time, which she seldom has. Whether for ten minutes or three hours, the important principle is that the student deserves the undivided attention of the instructor in a private, comfortable atmosphere if at all possible.

This means that the counselor or advisor cannot try to do several things at the same time, e.g. listening to a student, grading papers, answering the telephone, responding to other students' needs. The student may feel that you have only five minutes to spend with her, but she will respect this limit and accept it without difficulty *if* she has your undivided attention. Students dislike greatly the situation created when they come in to talk with a faculty member or counselor who is attempting to do a number of things at the same time. After a few tries they give up and go elsewhere. The advisor is much better off communicating, "Look, I'd very much like to talk with you, but I don't have

time right now; can we get together later on today at＿＿＿?" If either
of you is too busy at the moment to talk, don't try to see the student
to rush something through. It seldom works, and the resulting discouraged student is much less likely to return to you or to go and talk
with someone else. In general, then, the principle simply stated is that
whenever you are working with a student individually, or a class as a
group, she is the most important person in the world to you during that
time.

Once a relationship has been established—and this is a gradually developing process, not something that can be turned on and off—*the counselor can then begin to look at the problem* the student brings with her, and,
equally important, look at and see the student as a person. If information is necessary, the counselor and the student may gather it together, or the counselor may wish to gather certain information in order
to understand the nature of the problem more completely. The initial
approach depends to a great extent on the counselor's basic philosophy.
For example, in one school of counseling the counselor takes the lead
role in analyzing the problem, synthesizing all available information, and
diagnosing the problem and suggesting possible remedial actions. In
another school the emphasis is upon the student's taking the lead role
in these steps, the counselor acting as a catalyst. If we may use the
analogy of a medical setting, a patient comes in and says, "I don't feel
well." The physician establishes the relationship, and obtains the necessary information for a proper diagnosis. Once the diagnosis is reached,
either by the counselor, the counselee, or both, a course of action may
by recommended, or the student may be helped to see possible
alternatives open to her, and further assisted in reaching a decision herself on the most desirable course of action. A key point that should be
stressed here is that, as much as possible, we allow the student to determine her own rate of progress, i.e. the pace at which she will explore
her problem or reach a decision. In addition, we try to create conditions
that will allow the student to make her own decisions from her own
frame of reference.

But how can a counselor or faculty advisor know when a counseling
relationship has been established? This is difficult to assess. Certainly it
is not simply a matter of the student's continuing to come back. If we
try to look at the relationship from a student's point of view, there are
five key points which indicate that the foundation has been laid for a
sound counseling relationship.

1. *The student feels that someone has listened to her troubles. who cares about
her and has given her ego support.* The counselor may have done nothing
more than just listen to the student, but this is much easier said than
done. Typically, the student may have had these same problems on her
shoulders for a day or week or month without anybody with whom she
felt free to share her concerns. Now she feels that someone has really
listened to her, someone really cares, there is hope, and things are not
as black as she thought. One of the secrets of the truly empathic counselor is the ability to keep one's mouth shut and one's eyes and ears
open: the ability to be an empathic listener. Frequently the student

doesn't particularly need someone to tell her what to do, but rather she needs someone to listen to her as she explores her inner world.

2. *The student may have revealed what are to her horrible things in her life, yet the counselor continues to accept her rather than condemning her or judging her.* The student may have had the feeling, "I have done these terrible things. If I tell anyone about them, they will reject me, punish me or hurt me." Nevertheless the counselor continues to accept her, though she neither approves nor disapproves of the actions of the student. Even though the student has shared what are for her guilt-laden experiences, the counselor continues to accept her. As a result, the student begins to feel, "Maybe those things were not as bad as I thought—maybe I can learn to understand them, accept them, and live with them, after all."

3. *The student is relieved of her fears and doubts about entering the counseling situation.* This really refers back to the concept of rapport. When students first come in to talk to a counselor about personal concerns, they tend to be apprehensive and fearful. It is not easy for a student to open up, especially to a faculty advisor or a counselor with whom she has previously had a limited relationship. Consider yourselves: How easy would it be for you to walk in to someone in an authority position or someone whom you don't really know, and share your personal fears, concerns, and feelings of inadequacy? The student is made to feel that there is nothing to fear. "This person is human, as I am; this person cares about me enough to help, and this person will not use what I say to hurt me."

4. *The student can frequently gain greater insight by silence.* Remaining silent at times allows the counselor to listen more, and to be alert and sensitive to the nonverbal communication that is always present in the counseling session. Silence allows the counselee to continue to verbalize, and to think through her feelings and concerns.

5. *The student feels that something is being done by some plan,* even though it may be nothing more concrete than making another appointment. Although she has had this problem for some time without being able to solve it, she can begin to feel hope. "I can get help here." Coming back for another appointment for the student may be the beginning of working her way through the problem. For example, the student with feelings of inadequacy may want and need to explore these feelings. This will take time, but the student now has hope to keep her going; she feels better because she has finally taken concrete steps and action toward finding a solution or reaching greater self-understanding.

At this point let us examine the various kinds of faculty-student contacts that serve as an introduction to counseling.

## THE KIND OF CONTACT

There are many ways of counseling, ranging from a casual "on the fly" to a series of interviews over an extended period of time. Each may be initiated by either the faculty member or the student, and each has different characteristic features.

The first is the *casual counseling conversation*. This differs from a purely social conversation in that the student or the counselor has a specific purpose in mind. This casual counseling contact may take place in or out of class, in a clinical area, or a residence hall or cafeteria, almost anywhere that the faculty member and student come together. It is usually relatively brief, and occurs on no regular basis. It may be an opportunity for a student to ask an informational question or to relate her progress. It may also provide the counselor with the opportunity of making contact with the student in an informal manner to pave the way toward more formal contacts if the need arises. Care must be taken to try to maintain the confidentiality of these contacts, although this is usually difficult if not impossible because of the physical surroundings. In such a situation, if you find the student beginning to move into material better kept confidential, immediately suggest that you both move into a private area to continue the conversation, or try to make an appointment for the two of you to get together, preferably as soon as possible.

The second method is the *short-contact case*. One of the more common examples of this would be counseling and advising contacts which last 15 to 20 minutes. Again, these may be initiated by either the counselor or the student. In these short interviews, counselors try to help students with difficulties involving choice of courses or further education, failure in some phase of academic work, discipline problems, questions of a vocational nature—in short, areas that primarily require information giving. The counselor operates here as a resource, either providing information directly, or indicating sources where the information may be obtained. Such short time spans have been used for short-term psychotherapy, but in the context of nursing education such interviews will rarely delve into the personal-social areas. If these seem to be the main concern, the counselor is better off rescheduling another, more extensive appointment with the student. These relatively brief interviews are normally held in an office, ideally one that is private.

The other most common example of short-contact case may take several forms. In one form such a session is normally counselor-initiated for the purpose of orientation or problem identification, i.e. for teaching and diagnostic purposes. If this is the main purpose of the contact, then there are certain steps to follow to obtain the necessary data on which to base a decision:

a. What seems to be the derivation or source of the problem?
b. Is the nature of the need unique or does it follow a pattern?
c. Is the problem sporadic or chronic?
d. What is the extent of the need or problem—what effects does it have?
e. Is the problem diffused or clearly in focus?
f. How intense or severe does the problem seem?
g. In what form is the need or problem expressed?
h. What are the feelings that surround the need or problem?
i. How free is the student to deal with the need or problem?

Once these data have been gathered, the counselor is then ready to make a recommendation for action, or to help interpret the data to the student in a way that allows her to make an appropriate decision.

In its other form such a session is normally student-initiated. In either case the session usually lasts about 50 to 60 minutes. It is not recommended that sessions be longer than this, for even highly skilled and experienced counselors and therapists have found themselves unable to concentrate and be effective beyond this period of time. These sessions are not therapy sessions. They may be single contact or one of a series of such contacts. They are designed for the counselor to work with a normal student displaying the normal range of problems and concerns, which usually revolve around the personal-social area. In this sort of counseling the student is given time to think through her problem of development and adjustment in a permissive, accepting atmosphere.

The third method of counseling contact would be the *consultation service*. This is a much more highly structured service than the others. It usually follows a pattern of contacts which is distributed over several days or weeks. It normally consists of four or five parts: (*a*) The *intake or initial interview,* in which a counselor or interviewer determines the kind of service a student is seeking and describes the kinds of services the counselor can provide. (*b*) The *follow-up interview* with a counselor which usually occurs some days later, in which the student describes her interests, education, work experience, home conditions, recreation, future objectives, in short, anything that might be important and relevant to her and to the counselor. During this interview the counselor tries to sense the fundamental factors and concerns within the student. (*c*) The *testing period* with a psychometrist or psychologist in which necessary tests are given, and observations recorded of the student during testing. This stage will not always be a part of the consultation service; it depends upon the needs for additional information that might best be obtained through the use of tests. (*d*) *Case conferences* are held. Present are the counselor, usually the person who referred the student (another professional person), another experienced counselor for more objective reactions and the psychometrist or psychologist who administered the tests. In the case conference all available data on the student are collated and discussed, and interpretations are made as to the best course of action from this point on. (*e*) *Final interview,* in which the counselor gives the student the information she needs, interprets it, and encourages her to use the data in planning what seemed to the counselor to be the most feasible next step or alternative.

The final kind of counseling contact occurs in a group setting, and may be called *group guidance, group counseling,* or several other terms that are in current vogue such as sensitivity groups, encounter groups. Since our emphasis at this point is on one-to-one or individual counseling, these will be discussed in detail in Chapter 6.

## BEFORE THE SESSION BEGINS

Before a counselor and student sit down together to begin talking, several things must be taken into consideration. These are the set the counselor brings with her, the set the student brings with her, and the preparation for the session. Each is important and each will help to determine the success or failure of the counseling relationship.

1. **The Set of the Counselor.**   This occurs on both the conscious and the unconscious level. The unconscious set includes the value system, philosophy, personality, physical and psychological nature, and biases of the counselor. Some of these the counselor may be able to do little to change. It is vitally important, however, for the counselor to know herself, to know what causes her to act and react in certain situations. The conscious set normally includes the expectations a counselor brings to the session with her. For example, some counselors tend to get bored with educational-vocational counseling. If they believe that a student is coming in for career guidance, their lack of motivation may cause them to go through the motions, and at times miss hidden agenda, rather than recognizing the importance of a career decision to a student. Other counselors fall into the trap of believing that there is some pathologic state within every student. As a result, they push the student to talk about her "real" problem, rather than being able to accept the student as she presents herself.

The counselor is, above all, a human being. If she has learned to live with herself and accept herself, she is more likely to be able to accept other persons. If she is emotionally mature and feels fairly secure in her social and professional relations, she is able to help a less mature or less experienced person. The general attitude of the counselor is conveyed quickly to a student, through both verbal and nonverbal means. Thus the counselor cannot afford to be bored; she must allow sufficient time before each counseling session to get ready, to re-examine why the student is coming in, and to prepare herself physically and psychologically for the session.

2. **The Set of the Student Nurse.**   There are a number of factors which interrelate to affect the student as she comes to us. The counselor must be sensitive to these factors if she is to understand some of the dynamics that may be taking place, particularly in a first session with a student.

   a. The student's previous experience with counselors, and her psychological sophistication may be a positive influence for or provide resistance to counseling.
   b. If the student has been called in or sent in, she may not feel that she has a problem or may not be ready to accept any assistance.
   c. Students frequently come in very much afraid of the counselor, counseling, and themselves. They are particularly afraid of exposing too much of themselves, resulting in getting reduced or hurt by the unknown person with them. In simplest terms, students are very much afraid and resentful of being "psyched out" by a counselor or faculty member.
   d. Individuals in our society grow up believing that it is a sign of weakness if you cannot work out your problems for yourself, and must go to someone else for help. As a result, students sometimes come in convinced that they are "going crazy" or that there must be something drastically wrong with them.

3. **Preparation for the Session.**   Before a student is seen by a counselor, whether for a first or subsequent session, the counselor must do
some preparation. The amount depends somewhat on the counselor's
philosophy. Some of the more common steps to consider would include
the following:

   a. Availability of a private office that is comfortable, and which
      guarantees privacy, confidentiality, and relative quiet

   b. A desk that is clear so that the student doesn't feel that she is
      taking up too much of your time which is needed elsewhere

   c. Either a lock on the door or a clear understanding with a secretary
      that you are not to be disturbed

   d. An office arranged so that the desk is not placed between the
      counselor and the student as a physical as well as psychological
      barrier

   e. If appropriate, a review of the student's folder or previous
      session notes to refresh your memory as to who the student is, and
      why she may be coming in to see you. This must be done care-
      fully so as not to enter a session with a preconceived judgment as
      to the nature of the student's problem, or the desired specific
      actions to take

   f. Either no telephone or one that can be switched off or answered
      by a secretary outside.

Each of the foregoing steps is important to consider almost as a prerequisite checklist for a counselor. Adequate preparation may greatly
facilitate the development of a counseling relationship. Inadequate preparation may inhibit or kill the development of a counseling relationship
before it ever really gets started.

## OPENING THE COUNSELING SESSION

One of the most important aspects of the total counseling process
is the opening of a counseling session, regardless of the sort of counseling that is to be undertaken. Since the primary concern in the counseling relationship should eventually be self-understanding, and the ability
to self-determine necessary adjustments to cope with the problems
posed, then it is of the utmost importance that the relationship begin initially with a climate of warmth and acceptance. The problem of opening
a counseling session is often colored by events and situations completely
beyond the counselor's initial control. These relate to the kinds and
qualities of relationships previously established by the student, and in the
knowledge the counselor and student have of each other prior to the
initiation of the counseling relationship. If the relationship is biased by the
authoritarian or dogmatic role of the counselor who functions in other
roles within the school of nursing, then it is doubly important for her
to establish an acceptant attitude early in the counseling session. The student cannot feel free to express details of her personal concerns if she
feels that moral, ethical, and value judgments will be made by the counselor.

The oversolicitous counselor can be as much a threat to the student as the one who maintains an air of complete indifference to the relationship, the concerns expressed, or the student. We must assume that if the student has taken the time and energy to refer herself to a counselor for assistance, then the problem with which she is concerned is a serious one to her, and deserves full acceptance by the counselor. But acceptance is not merely being physically in the counseling session, or the nodding of one's head in approval; it is a feeling of acceptance, understanding, and involvement that is communicated verbally and nonverbally by the counselor from the very first contact with the student.

Let us for the moment examine a hypothetical situation in which a student nurse asks to talk with one of her clinical instructors. For one or more reasons the clinical instructor has previously had occasion to reprimand the student. After the initial greeting the student, acting as a counselee in this situation, states that she is having some difficulty with a particular phase of her program. The initial reaction of the counselor will in fact structure the counseling relationship until some subsequent act or statement alters it. For example, let us suppose that the initial reaction of the counselor is, "I am not in the least surprised at your difficulty, since the reports that have come to me and my observations have indicated that you seem to be consistently inattentive and disinterested." Needless to say there are many busy, harried faculty members whose reaction might be similar to this. Such a response has the potential effect of making the student angry and defensive, attitudes hardly conducive to the start of a helping relationship. If you are to serve in the role of a counselor, you must indicate by your initial reaction that you are interested, concerned, and ready to listen to the student's problem.

There are no magic ways to start a conference, interview or counseling session. Each is dependent upon the individual circumstances and situation. Some students will enter the counseling session with hidden desires to be told what to do; others are seeking assistance in thinking through a situation or concern, still others have already decided what they want to do, and are looking to the counselor for approval or confirmation. Students sometimes need to start a counseling session with another problem than the one which is really bothering them. Others consciously leave out relevant details, or misrepresent their problems until they feel comfortable enough and are given the opportunity to clarify later.

The first statement after the initial greeting may be the most important one made by the counselor. There are some useful things to remember about such a statement.

1. It should help to put the student at ease, and can occur with any kind of warm, accepting greeting.

2. The first statement can and often does set the stage for the beginning of the counseling session.

3. Students will enter a session with many kinds of problems and varying frames of mind. A disarming statement such as "You seem to have something on your mind; would you like to tell me about it," will often help to start a session. Other such accepting statements might be, "You asked to see me?" or, "How can I help you?"

4. The tone of voice and inflection used by the counselor in speaking are of utmost importance. Calm and relaxed moods are guidelines.

5. The counselor's involvement from this point on will be somewhat dependent on the readiness of the student to begin a session. If the counselor has asked the student to come in, she should make an initial encouraging statement and then remain silent, allow the student to talk, and concentrate on listening and understanding.

6. A big smile and relaxed attitude may at times seem out of place to a student who feels that her problem is a serious one for her.

7. The main emphasis in beginning a counseling session should be to give the impression that you are willing to listen and genuinely want to help.

## DURING THE COUNSELING SESSION

During the interview the counselor encourages the student to think through her problems, and to develop a positive self-concept. She listens to the student as though nothing else in the world were more important to her. Indeed, whether a session is five or 50 minutes, students appreciate greatly that, no matter how busy you may be, when you are with them they are of primary importance to you. This intentness is necessary if the counselor is really to understand the student. The counselor tries to see the student in three ways: as she sees herself, as she really is, and as she would like to be and can become.

With such fundamental respect for other people, the counselor naturally will not force her ideas on the student, nor insist that she conform to the counselor's values, standards or morals. She recognizes inherent differences between her own cultural background and that of the student. For example, parents' ideas about what their children should do or be may be very different from those of the counselor. The counselor will always acknowledge the validity of another's way of life. She will encourage the student to express her thoughts and feelings freely and to take all possible initiative and responsibility for her own growth. She must not be concerned with maintaining school and college standards at the expense of helping the student make the wisest decisions for her.

The process of counseling is a constantly changing and evolving one, but we are often conditioned to respond in the same manner as to previous experiences from other counseling sessions. There are several extremes of responses that the counselor should attempt to avoid. These include the following:

1. *Overemphasis or underemphasis*—placing too much or too little importance on a statement or idea or action by the student

2. *Overanticipation or underanticipation*—prejudging what the student is going to say before she says it, or being totally surprised by the unexpected nature of the student's disclosures

3. *Overaccepting or underaccepting*—blind acceptance of everything the student says or does, or selective rejection of what the student may say or do

4. *Overexcusing or underexcusing*—rationalizing or justifying actions or

statements by the student, or failing to recognize the validity for the student of some of his excuses

5. *Being oversolicitous or undersolicitous*—being so concerned that you suffocate the student in sympathy, or remaining so distant and objective that you are seen as cold and impersonal.

Counseling involves the constant interaction of two distinct personalities, but the personality of the counselor must adjust to that of the student. Some students do not necessarily want to be accepted by the counselor as a personality or to be psychoanalyzed, but merely wish assistance in working through their concern. The counselor to them is a professional who can help deal with their concern. The student is also not necessarily looking for a friend. Another extreme in a counseling session is stressing the *I*, the counselor, rather than *you*, the student. When asking a direct question, some counselors will bring the weight of their status and position to bear so that they can answer as an authority. This procedure may make the counselor feel good, but often will not help the student, who is so overwhelmed by the authority of the statement that she is unable to challenge and think through the best alternatives for her.

Another important point in a counseling session revolves around recording a session or taking notes during it. No session should ever be recorded without the knowledge and permission of the student. If you desire to record a session (an excellent way to check on and improve your own counseling skills), a possible way to obtain such permission may be, "Frequently I try to record my sessions with students. When I do, I don't have to take any notes during the session and can concentrate on you and what you are saying. It also allows me to go back over the tape later to see if there are things that I missed which may enable me to be of more help to you. Such tapes of course are completely confidential. If you feel the tape recorder won't be in our way, I thought we might use it today. If at any point you feel that it is interfering with our session, please let me know and I will shut it off. Also, if at any time you wish to hear the tape of a session, we can play it together here before the tape is erased. How does that sound to you?"

Taking notes during a session or bringing a student folder with you into a counseling session creates barriers to communication. It is impossible to talk and listen and write at the same time. If you have a folder with the name of the student on it, inevitably she begins to wonder what is in there. If you take notes, the student becomes anxious to know what you are writing down. If you must take notes, however, you can explain the rationale and operate as in the example cited above.

Either way, the notes or folder interferes with rather than enhances the development of a sound relationship. If you need specific sheets from a folder for informational purposes, it would be better to bring the information with you, and place it on the table or desk near you so that the student can easily see and read them. If you are not recording a session, it is better to sit down immediately after a session either to write up what happened while it is fresh in your mind, or at least to make some notes or dictation that will allow you to write up the session later in the day. In general, sessions should be written up the same day, or they begin to blur together and lose some of their relevancy.

## CLOSING THE COUNSELING SESSION

Closing a counseling session may be a simple procedure if a natural break occurs, or quite difficult if one does not occur. If no time limit has been set on the session (we have already mentioned that the normal maximum for a session is about 50 minutes), students will occasionally go on indefinitely. If the student is emotionally upset, it is desirable to give her a few minutes to pull herself together before she leaves. But rarely is it either useful or practical to prolong a session more than an hour. How a counseling session concludes may have a vital bearing on the future success of the counseling relationship, including whether or not the student comes back.

If the counselor wishes to terminate the session, any of the following may be used, depending on the nature of the relationship.

1. The counselor may summarize what has been covered in the session to indicate progress and understanding, and to pave the way for the next session. "We have covered a great deal today that helps me understand how you feel. We talked about . . . . It seems that you have already given this a great deal of thought. Why don't we continue this next time?"

2. The counselor may give the student something concrete to do or to take with her for the next session. "From what you have said, it would seem useful for you to talk to your pediatrics instructor. If you can do that before we get together next time, we can then talk about what you have found out."Or, "Your questions about careers in nursing following graduation are good ones. I have some material here on possible careers that you can take with you to read, and we can talk about your reactions next time."

3. If the student shows no signs of leaving or terminating the session, the counselor may say, "I see our time is almost up for today." She can then give the student a few minutes before announcing that the time is up. Occasionally the counselor may have to stand up and escort the student to the door before she really gets the message. If a student continues to talk even with the door open, the counselor should acknowledge what is being said, but not prolong the session. Instead, she should reinforce the idea of continuing at the next session. In the following session the counselor may wish to explore the student's feelings about having to leave the counseling session before she may have felt ready.

Some students seem to be more comfortable operating in a "hit and run" situation—they drop an emotional bomb by bringing up what is for them a threatening area, and then quickly leave. This can be quite frustrating to a counselor, who is left wondering what to do. One possibility would be to call the student back to see if she wishes to talk further. If not, the counselor should make clear that she will be available if the student feels the need to talk. Another more likely approach would be to bring up the subject early in the next session and try to help the student deal with it.

If the student terminates the session abruptly, or at the close of an hour, any of the following may appropriately be used.

1. The counselor might suggest that the student make another appointment at her convenience if she feels the need for additional assistance or information.

2. The counselor might suggest a specific time and date for the student to return. If the student does not wish to make another appointment, the counselor may say, "I can understand that you may not feel like making another appointment right now. However, I think it would be useful to you if we could talk some more. I'll set aside time next Tuesday at 10:00. I'll be here if you decide to come in. I hope you will."

3. The counselor might allow the student to leave without saying anything, assuming that she will return of her own volition, or that informal contacts may pave the way for her return at a later time.

4. In the extremely rare case of a student who, in the counselor's judgment, cannot safely be allowed to leave, she should be taken to the health center or some other place where she can receive appropriate medical or psychiatric assistance.

5. In the event a referral is indicated, the counselor should usually take the initiative in introducing the idea. This situation will be discussed in detail in Chapter 7.

It must be remembered that any of the suggested statements given here are just that—suggestions. In the final analysis, the best response usually comes from the sensitivity and understanding of the counselor. It also must be stressed once again that we view students as basically normal human beings, rather than fragile, abnormal and without resources or abilities. Therefore the counselor must always keep in mind the autonomy, the insight, and the capacity for self-development in the student. The more the counselor can respect these qualities in the student, the more helpful she will be.

## FOLLOWING THE SESSION

After a session is over the relationship continues. Both the counselor and the student carry the effects of the session away with them. The counselor may:

1. As soon as possible write or dictate whatever notes she wishes to maintain of the counseling session.
2. Start to get ready for the next appointment by following the same preparatory steps previously recommended.
3. Consult with other professionals about the concerns expressed in a particular situation. Caution must always be exercised in maintaining confidentiality.

A student may:

1. Continue to think about what has been discussed during the session, including sharing the ideas expressed with others.
2. Reject you as a counselor completely in the future if she has revealed intimate details not previously disclosed to anyone else. Rarely, a student may feel ashamed or may feel that she said much

more than she intended. In such a situation any attempt at re-establishing a counseling relationship by a counselor will be difficult or completely rejected. The counselor must be able to accept this position by the student.

3. Follow through on the suggestions for action prior to the next appointment.

## SUMMARY

A counseling session is a dynamic, living process with an infinite variety of outcomes. Just as there is no single right way to counsel, there is no magic formula or series of steps that will ensure the smooth development of a counseling relationship. Nevertheless, if the faculty member remembers the points that have been covered in these first three chapters, she is on the road toward operating as a counseling professional. These points include:

1. Following the ethical standards of counseling
2. Knowing who she is and how she acts, reacts, and interacts with fellow human beings
3. Doing a satisfactory job of preparing for a counseling session
4. Working with the student to diagnose the problem
5. Accepting the problem presented by the student, and the student herself
6. Working with the student to plan a course of action
7. Reinforcing positive actions by the student
8. Following up a session with additional sessions if needed, or with informal contacts
9. Reinforcing the availability of assistance if needed in the future
10. Above all, recognizing that the student has the capacity within her to make the best decisions for her, and recognizing even more that the counselor is not God and cannot be all things to all men.

There are counselors who occasionally succumb to the trap of falling victim to a messianic complex, i.e. believing that they must save the world and that all decisions and responsibility rest on their shoulders. This denies the fact that whatever a student does or becomes may (a) be due in part to the positive or negative influence of the counselor; (b) have little or no relation to the work of the counselor, but be a result of a change in environmental stress. As counselors, we cannot be equally successful with all students, nor is the responsibility solely ours for a student's decisions. It is usually difficult to define counseling success or assess the effectiveness of counseling. For this reason, counseling is probably the wrong profession or activity for those faculty members who need constant reassuring evidence of the success of their work.

# Chapter 4

# Counselee Needs and Concerns

We have described some of the characteristics of the counseling relationship, and points for the faculty member to consider before, during, and after a counseling session. At this point it is time to turn to the other half of the relationship, i.e. the student nurse. In so doing, we are faced with the same areas of student difficulty as normally occur in higher education. Thus we need to look at who should be counseled, what are the signs that counseling may not be working successfully, and some general observations on student behavior. In addition, it is necessary to take a close look at a large problem area among students in higher education, i.e. attitudes toward and addiction to various forms of drugs.

## WHO SHOULD BE COUNSELED

It should be emphasized at this point that the purpose of counseling is not to provide long-term therapy for students. Such exceptional cases almost invariably require referral. Rather, counseling services should be designed to remove some of the barriers that interfere with a student's performance or ability to learn. Or to phrase it another way, we are working with an essentially normal student who may be reacting to a particularly abnormal situation in a very normal way. By assisting her to work through some of her concerns, it is possible to help her become a happier person, a more productive human being, and a nurse with much greater sensitivity to the personal needs of the patients for whom she is providing care.

There are some general situations in which counseling may be indicated as useful. These situations revolve around at least five groups of students.

The first of these would be the *marginal student*. We are referring here to the student nurse who has demonstrated the necessary ability for admission to the school of nursing, but is functioning at a level below average. Do we identify early those students whose previous performance and predictive score would seem to indicate good work, but are achieving far below their indicated ability? Do we try to explore with such students the reasons behind the marginal achievement? Do we try to aid each student in reaching a proper understanding of her capabilities? Is the student helped when necessary to explore and establish acceptable (to her) alternative goals? Does the student who can't quite make it through your program quietly disappear, or is some effort made through counseling and exit interviews to help her find other directions that are useful and desirable to her?

There are a variety of reasons why a student underachieves, including poor motivation, personal problems, poor study habits, interference from outside sources, excessive competition, and others. Some of these can be worked through by a counselor working with the student. If assistance is not successful, in too many cases in schools and colleges the student who fails quietly disappears, unmourned and unmissed. As educational institutions, schools have a responsibility to all students once they are admitted to help each one make the best possible adjustment within the school, and, if they fail, to help them find acceptable, wise alternatives.

The second group is comprised of the *superior students*. Do we identify such students early? Do we provide a program for their full development? In other words, have we built a lock-step curriculum so that superior students are neither encouraged nor permitted to work up to their ability and go on? Have we been teaching for the middle group, ignoring the needs of those students at either end? When we recognize superior ability, and see that the student is not achieving at the level of her potential, do we try to provide counseling to find out why, and attempt to alleviate the problem?

The third group consists of those students with *behavioral problems*. Do we concentrate our efforts on forcing our acting-out students to behave and conform, or do we try to understand their behavior and the underlying reasons for it? Is the acting-out behavior generic within the total student group, or specific with one or more individuals? What within our program fosters antisocial behavior? Some readers may recall the study reported in *Transaction* several years ago which compared acting-out student nurses with student leaders among the same group of students. The study indicated that the so-called trouble-makers were consistently rated higher as graduate nurses in terms of creativity, leadership, initiative, and so on, than those who were leaders as students. This may indicate something about the nature of our schools and colleges. Perhaps we encourage leadership among those who conform to our expectations and "follow the party line." Counseling may help us assist the behavioral problem student to utilize her talents in ways that are more constructive for her. In any event, we need to be sure that our student government is representative of all students, rather than just the "good" ones.

The fourth group is made up of the *culturally different* students. What provisions do we make for students whose cultural, ethnic, sexual make-up is different from that of the majority of students within the school of nursing? If the majority are white or female or young, for example, do we make an effort through programs or through counseling to help the black, the male or the older student to be accepted within the larger group of students? Nursing as a profession has been making a strong effort to recruit men and blacks into the field. Do we stop at recruitment, or do we recognize the differences among students in building our program? This group will be discussed in a little more detail in the next chapter.

The final group that presents a concern to us would include those students who don't belong, i.e. the loner, the social misfit, the young man or woman who somehow never seems to fit in with the rest of the student body. It is not uncommon for such students to be equally avoided by faculty members. Do we make an effort to identify such students so as, among other things, to help us separate the loners from the lonely? Do we try to offer counseling assistance to these students to try to aid them to better understand and accept themselves, and ultimately to help them find a useful, satisfying place for themselves within the school and within society? This is the group that is most frequently overlooked and unaided. Yet it may be composed of individual students who need our help the most.

## DRUGS AND THE NURSING STUDENT

There is a growing apprehension among nursing educators that students will enter their academic and clinical programs with a greater proclivity for drug abuse than may be found among college students in general. At present, however, no one really knows how extensive drug abuse by student nurses is. We do know that the problems of drug use and abuse are on the upswing in all segments of our society. It is also significant that most studies report that drug abusers have their first drug experience while in their teens. This could mean that many of the drug-abusing students will have brought their problem with them into the school of nursing. Thus we have the concern among nursing educators about problems of drugs, identification of drug abuse, emergency care for drug abuse, and professional concerns about student nurses and drugs.

Nursing educators are for the most part nurses, professionals who over time have acquired their own fears, prejudices, and sometimes contempt, for the patient who has abused drugs, or sought to abuse them while hospitalized for various illnesses. They are all too familiar with postoperative and other kinds of patients who maintain symptoms, pains, and analgesic demands disproportionate with a true pathologic state. These patients soon take on the image of being weak and demanding, and may ultimately be labeled as "addicts" and charted as such. As a result, nurses may at times withhold medication when there is a legitimate need for fear that the patient will become an addict. Sometimes these patients simply are not liked by nursing personnel, sometimes to the point of contempt, depending on the feelings aroused in the nurse. Thus the nursing educator, leaving the field of clinical practice and entering that of education, may have already acquired an attitude about drugs and those who use them. This attitude, expectancy or "set" can be a serious obstacle to her being an effective resource with her students in both the preventive and interventive teaching and counseling roles that she will encounter in the fulfillment of her responsibilities to her students.

Thus we have the nursing educator of today facing two significant barriers to her ability to work effectively with drug abuse problems among her students. First, she may be aware that many of her students will have experienced drug use or abuse before entering the school of nursing. Second, her own perceptions and convictions, and those of society, about drug abuse could be distorted to the point at which she finds it difficult to shed her own experiences and prejudices, and thus be unable to relate to or respond to the drug problems that may arise among her students. Will she see these students in the same way as society sees them or as she perceived former patients, or will she see them as persons in need of help rather than punishment; as potentially strong persons if only because they may have been able to trust the faculty member to whom they disclose their fears and problems with drugs?

If it be true that student nurses present us with the fear of proclivity to drug abuse simply because they are members of what we call the "youth generation," and "drugs are part of youth today," then what can the nursing educator do for this segment of youth that seeks personal and professional growth and fulfillment in the nursing profession?

Realistically, the student nurse would be most hesitant about seeking help from faculty members about drugs. Given the traditional and current convictions and regulations about drug abuse in nursing education, the student nurse would in all probability bring her problem to a counselor or someone else with whom for one reason or another she has established trust, rapport, and, most importantly, acceptance as a person. Current nursing educational programs would make it risky for the student nurse to reveal drug problems to a faculty member, because the student would perceive herself as exposed to a punitive response, with a strong likelihood of dismissal from the nursing program.

It seems appropriate at this point to clarify for the nursing educator the kinds of drug abuse her students may have been exposed to or participated in before entrance into the nursing program. The adolescent drug abuser will usually fall into one of three categories. Curiosity and peer competition are the principal precipitators of the first category, *"the taster."* This would refer to the person who has used drugs in peer social settings because she is curious, and because she is expected to join the crowd as they experiment.

Almost invariably the first, and often the only, drug abused is marijuana. Current research would indicate that this is a drug of little if any toxicity, and is not prone to precipitate dependency, either physiological or psychological. This drug is generally dangerous to the user not because of its chemical constituents, but because of how it is prepared. Because of its relative impotency as a stimulant or producer of a euphoric reaction, it has often been "cut" with or strengthened with other chemicals to make it more acceptable to the user, and thus more profitable to the seller. Current additives are strychnine and, most recently, formic acid to add to its psychophysiological effect for the user. Because it is usually smoked, it requires an effective burning mixture. Dried and strained rat droppings have been found to be effective as a compatible burning agent to produce a longer, more effective smoke. Needless to say, the toxicity of this reagent, which is heavily laden with bacteria, would sharply increase the risk to the user, and is of more concern than the drug itself. The "taster" may have been exposed to a few other drugs such as LSD and the amphetamines. Again, the use is usually motivated by curiosity and peer competition.

It would seem that the psychosocial development of the adolescent "taster" is the prime factor that limits her use to a few experiences with drugs, and eventually her complete discontinuance of them. She simply doesn't need them, her curiosity has been satisfied, and her peer demands are no longer sufficiently relevant for her to continue on these drugs, or to proceed to the second stage, that of the *"drug chaser."*

This person is one who has tried drugs of the weaker variety, and found them to be enjoyable to the extent that she will rather consistently seek and use them, not in an addictive manner, but because of her high dependency on peer acceptance and the "escape from reality" that such drugs bestow upon her. The "chaser" shifts from the use of marijuana to the amphetamines, hallucinogens, barbiturates, and sometimes to the hard narcotics, especially heroin and other morphine derivatives, thereby increasing her proclivity to physiological as well as psychological addiction.

The third category of drug abuser has often been called the *"head."* This is the person who has converted her entire life style to obtaining and using drugs of abuse on a daily basis. She is obsessed with this need as her way of coping with the reality of life around her that she perceives to be entirely alien and threatening to her. She actively resents traditional societal values and practices and builds her own world of euphoria, delusions, and hallucinations. Most of her lucid periods of awareness are devoted to finding means to maintain her artificial world.

The third category of drug abuser, the "head," will seldom present problems for nursing educators because the likelihood of such persons being interested in pursuing the profession of nursing would be minimal. The academic, financial, and social conditions of a nursing program would be outside their choice of priorities in their artificial world. They have only one priority, i.e. obtaining the means to and the use of all varieties of drugs, hallucinogens, stimulants, and hard narcotics.

What are the implications for nursing educators of the other two kinds of drug users? The first category, the "taster," would not seem to present problems to faculty members in her ability to meet academic and clinical expectations. Quite the contrary, the ability to be a "taster" only, with subsequent cessation of drug use, would indicate a relatively high degree of maturity. Such students have found more appropriate methods for coping with stress and peer competition; they neither want nor need drugs to sustain them in the face of conflict and stress. The second category, the "chaser," does present a problem and a potentially high risk in the nursing profession. She has found a need for drug abuse, for her drugs are effective as coping reactions. Although inappropriate, they nevertheless become the means of choice when the student nurse is confronted with conflict, stress, and a need to escape. Given the accessibility to drugs in a hospital setting, this student would be a likely candidate for future addiction.

As we mentioned, the principal category of drug abuse problems to be faced by nursing educators will be the group known as the "chaser." She will be a person usually high in dependency needs, rather immature and irresponsible, and often hostile toward traditional educational programs. This person will have learned effective means of deception for meeting her drug needs even before entering the school of nursing and the clinical setting. She may find it extremely difficult to cope with the new life style expected of a student nurse, the academic and professional expectancies of the nursing profession, the rules and regulations newly imposed upon her, and, for the student in a hospital school of nursing, the semisegregated living conditions.

Such a person would not hesitate to use amphetamines as a necessary stimulant to maintaining academic requirements, long hours of study, and personal and professional expectations. She has learned how to obtain and use drugs in the past; given the new stress situation in the school of nursing, she will likely renew the use of these drugs. In addition, students with no prior experience with drugs may find it difficult to resist the temptation under the same stress.

### Identification of Drug Abuse

Common symptoms of drug abuse are nonexistent. Dramatic changes in a student's attitude and behavior *may* be a gross method of suspecting drug abuse. Signs which might suggest drug abuse would be sudden and dramatic change in attendance, alertness, reaction to authority, and significantly altered academic performance. Another possible symptom may be unusual degrees of activity or inactivity. In most cases, however, it is difficult to determine whether drug abuse precipitated dramatic behavioral change, whether dramatic change precipitated drug abuse, or whether the dramatic change in behavior reflects simply changes in the student's environment which are not drug-related.

The *depressant* drug abuser, using such drugs as barbiturates or certain tranquilizers, exhibits most of the symptoms of alcohol intoxication with one important difference: there is no odor of alcohol. The greatest hazard with depressants would be overdose or acute toxic reaction, which could result in the critical impairment of life signs and possibly death.

The *stimulant* abuser most commonly uses amphetamines and related mood-elevating drugs. Drug influence is characterized by excessive activity, a sense of power, and overconfidence. The stimulant abuser is easily aroused to anger, is irritable, argumentative, and extremely nervous. Pupillary dilation may be present even in bright light. A dry mouth and nose and bad breath are also prevalent accompanying signs.

The *hallucinogenic* abuser is most likely to use a drug such as LSD outside of the school or hospital setting. These drugs are usually taken in a group or social situation where there are special conditions designed to enhance the dream or trancelike effect of the drug, such as the use of music and lights. The effect of these drugs is not always euphoric; on occasion, users can experience negative effects such as terrifying nightmares and sporadic remissions without the intake of additional drugs.

The *marijuana* user is most difficult to identify unless directly under the influence of a hallucinogenic high. Marijuana acts similar to stimulant drugs on the upswing of the drug effect, and then acts as a depressant on the downswing, often leaving the user in a stuporous or sleepy state. The effect varies greatly, depending on the user's prior mood and external surroundings. Controversy currently surrounds the negative, habituating effects of the drug, if any. No evidence to date clearly delineates what, if any, long-term debilitative effects marijuana has on the user.

*Alcohol* abusers show a high frequency of drug use on a spree or thrill basis. It is a more socially acceptable drug which can have significant retardant effects on psychomotor ability and judgment.

The principal concern in dealing with drug toxicity or overdose is the identification of the drug, its strength, purity, and effect on the abuser without laboratory tests. Another concern is the multiple forms in which the drug can be found. A third concern revolves around the fact that abusers may mix several kinds of drugs at one time, a fact which greatly compounds both the effects and the problems. Finally, we must recognize that students will occasionally find themselves under the influence of drugs without knowing it; i.e. they have taken or been given something accidentally without realizing that it was a drug. This may become especially frightening to a student, for she is unable to account for her behavior.

## Emergency Care for Drug Abuse

The nursing educator, as well as the fellow nursing student, may be called upon without notice to aid a student experiencing negative drug effects, toxic overdose, and postdrug effects such as psychotic episodes. Students and faculty should be well informed on emergency procedures to be used. These may include physician coverage, the use of emergency room facilities and equipment, and the presence of someone who can provide reassurance and assistance to the student while she is experiencing the drug effect. The main concern is to protect the student from injury and to minimize emotional trauma. If the student is on depressants or "downs," the objective is to assist the student to maintain normal life signs through administration of counteracting medications or use of respirators, stomach pumps, and so forth, as a significant first step. This should be followed by reassurance and support of the student as she endures the drug effects.

Most drug reactions involving hallucinogenic drugs will not require emergency medical intervention. If the student is on a bad "acid" trip, all counteracting drugs may be contraindicated because of the uncertainty of what was taken. Also, stomach pumps and the like will not take drugs such as LSD and mescaline out of the system. Referral resources which will allow the student to come down from the effects of drugs in a protective, supportive fashion may lessen the negative effects of the drug reaction. Drug abuse centers which can provide reliable and competent care for the student should be identified and made known to both students and faculty. In every instance it is recommended that such a center be utilized when possible to deal with emergencies.

Although most medically supervised drug abuse centers are able to deal with detoxification, few are able to provide adequate therapy or counseling. The added fear of involvement with legal authorities causes drug abusers to seek out nonmedical lay help.

In response to the need for lay help, many educational institutions have found developing around them drug information centers, "hot lines," drop-in centers, and the like. These organizations and centers are usually staffed by nonprofessionals who have had some training or experience with the effects of drugs. Although these centers may lack professionally trained staff, they do provide the supportive and protective elements. It would be advisable for faculty members to get to know these resources, since many of the students find them less threatening than more formalized treatment centers. Many of these centers are gaining professional support and community acceptance, and therefore are approaching the ability to provide comprehensive drug abuse treatment.

In a study done by student nurse members of a district association in Ohio, 151 student nurses were surveyed on attitudes toward drug abuse. In the results, 74 per cent approved of the establishment of methadone clinics as a form of rehabilitation for heroin addicts; 77 per cent were opposed to legalization of the use of marijuana; 94 per cent were in favor of the establishment of drug clinics to help drug addicts who come in on their own. Such addicts are not reported to the police. Students felt that this was effective therapy. Sixty-one per cent felt that kids take drugs for kicks, and 85 per cent felt that drug use is a symptom of deeper emotional problems. When asked what they, as student nurses, could do to help solve the drug problem, some of the suggestions included getting involved in rehabilitation both through school courses and volunteer work, supporting legislation and encouraging the development of walk-in clinics, and setting a good example. Essentially, they felt that more people are needed who are willing to listen and be nonjudgmental to those desiring help.

### Professional Concerns About Drug Abuse

If drug abuse is confirmed, the nursing educator is faced with an ethical as well as a legal problem. Most schools of nursing have codes of conduct, as does the profession of nursing. Of particular importance is a well thought out ethical stand in dealing with drug abuse within each school of nursing. The nursing faculty must also consider the legal implications, as well as the rights of the student and her professional potential in contrast with the degree of severity of the abuse. Whatever the code of conduct and the ethical stand of the faculty on drug use and abuse, the student body should be given full and accurate information about the position of the faculty and the school of nursing.

Student drug abusers may lose their opportunity to engage in a career in nursing because of immediate dismissal if caught. Although little argument would be encountered in the automatic dismissal of a blatant, hard-core user, there is concern for the appropriateness of dismissing the spree user. One could argue that students engaged in thrill seeking through drugs are clearly demonstrating irresponsible and immature behavior which could seriously hamper their ability to function as competent nurses. Whether or not a student is using drugs, it would seem that the main concern of the faculty should be the student's ability to function in a responsible, competent manner. It may be wiser to examine the drug abuse in the context of the total individual, in that drug abuse may be one of many signs which indicate suitability or unsuitability for nursing. It's worth noting that dismissal does not really cope with the problem.

The nursing educator who is involved as teacher and counselor to her students would be well advised to undertake the following considerations. The nursing educator should be aware that the statistics on adolescent drug abuse are highly unreliable, as are the nature and functions of the more commonly used hallucinogens. The illegal status of these drugs has made it extremely difficult to assess both their use and their psychophysiological effects. At present there is only one institution in the United States allowed human experimentation with marijuana, and another permitted to do research on LSD, mescaline, and psilocybin, the three most potent and common hallucinogens, other than marijuana.

The nursing educator, whether in didactic presentations about drugs of abuse, or in a counseling relationship with a student, must give first priority to attaining accurate knowledge of all these drugs in all their aspects and communicating this knowledge clearly to students. This includes not only their properties of absorption, biotransformation, and systemic distribution, but also, more importantly, what motivates their use, the common personality traits of the "chaser," and more in-depth knowledge of the social as well as the psychophysiological ingredients of drug abuse. There is nothing so effective in building distrust and lack of credibility in the drug abuser than inaccurate, myth-laden presentations on drug abuse, whether in the classroom or the faculty member's office when she is called upon for help by a student.

What is even more destructive in a faculty-student relationship is the often unconscious suspicion of the faculty member communicated to the student. This manifests itself in the "pupil peekers," i.e. faculty members and medical personnel who look for pupillary reactions such as vasoconstriction or dilation that might signal the observer that this student is on drugs. Many students have been exposed to this type of "diagnosis" in their homes and school settings, and it screams out the most destructive counselor-student message, i.e. *distrust*. Such ocular vasoconstriction or dilation more often than not may be a function of stressful reading or too many hours watching television. It should be clearly emphasized at this point that knowledge of drug signs without knowledge of the student may be disastrous to a possible productive, helping relationship.

As nursing educators, you should assume that most of your students have not been and are not now involved in drug abuse. The nursing educator who re-assesses her own attitudes toward drug abuse, who takes a leadership role in changing academic systems that contribute to unnecessary conflicts and stresses that trigger drug abuse, who responds to each student in need with trust and acceptance, will find it more comfortable to be both a teacher and a counselor to her students.

## PROBLEMS IN THE COUNSELING RELATIONSHIP

There are times when any counselor, no matter how experienced, begins to wonder about her effectiveness in a particular counseling relationship. We have already mentioned that counselors are not equally effective with all students with whom they come in contact. Success in a counseling relationship is an ambiguous term that is usually determined differently by each counselor. Some criteria used are changed behavior, change in grades or performance, and statements by the student after counseling. Nevertheless the counselor who attempts to measure her effectiveness by the "success" or "failure" of each student with whom she worked will soon find herself ruled by her emotions. This represents an emotional luxury which counselors can ill afford.

There are also times when the counselor begins to wonder about the effects of the help she offered to a student. If the student fails to follow the advice given or the decision agreed upon, the counselor may feel that she has wasted her efforts and failed. If the student follows the advice given or the plan agreed upon, any resulting tragedies may be viewed by the counselor as her responsibility resulting from her inability to make the kinds of suggestions that would help the student solve her problems. This ignores the point made earlier that the student may have lacked the ability to follow through and solve her own problems. Unfortunately, the counselor, being human, is concerned about her own adequacy as a helping individual, and therefore is vulnerable and potentially less effective.

It is important for a faculty member doing counseling to begin to recognize problems in the counseling relationship. There are several situations that may indicate to the counselor the need for termination, referral or, at the very least, a careful discussion with the student.

The first problem that occurs is *the development of a sense of dependency*. Occasionally a student may come to lean heavily upon you for advice and decision making. Transference may also occur in some situations. You must be alert to this possibility, and not become too disturbed if it occurs. A compounding problem that occurs is when the counselor also begins to find this relationship a personally satisfying one. As counselors, we must realize that we cannot live others' lives for them, and that the criterion of the successful counseling relationship is the gradually evolving ability of the student to stand on her own two feet, and to be able to break off the counseling relationship when appropriate. It is of course possible that close friendship may be established over a period of time between a faculty member and a student. The problem in such a situation lies in determining whether, in fact, a long-standing relationship is one of friendship, as opposed to one of dependency. This, at times, is a difficult discrimination to make.

A second problem revolves around *irregular appointments*. The student who fails to show up when she is expected, or who cancels appointments often, is telling you something. She may be telling you that the material presently being discussed is of such a threatening nature that she cannot bring herself to continue the discussion at this point. She may be saying that she does not feel that the counseling experience is helping her. Other less common possibilities include the student's desire to punish the counselor or someone else significant in her life, or extreme disorganization. The counselor needs to ask herself whether these irregularities are noticed in many students. If they are, inadequate counseling procedures seem to be indicated. More often, however, only a few students display this behavior, and, as annoying as it may be, it provides another symptom of maladjustment to be weighed along with other behavioral symptoms displayed by an individual student.

The third problem occurs in the case of a *personality clash* between the faculty member and the student. It has been mentioned before that no one can be a counselor to all people. Just as some proportion of failure is built into the counseling process, so is a certain proportion of misfits between the personality patterns of the faculty member and those of the student. When you discover that you don't like a student or that she doesn't like you, a first step may be to discuss the difficulty with a colleague. Perhaps your own perception is distorted. If, however, you are unable to effect a change in your attitude or the student's, a counseling relationship is probably impossible between the two of you. In such cases, referral is indicated at the earliest opportunity. The advantage of an early referral is that the student gets better assistance sooner, and you may avoid having her develop a negative attitude toward counseling and counselors in general which will prevent her from seeking appropriate help in the future.

A fourth problem revolves around *the use of defense mechanisms*. Most nursing educators are familiar with the literature on defense mechanisms. Rationalization, compensation, projection, reaction formation, and so on, are all terms used to describe techniques used by the individual to avoid catastrophic experiences, to make life more bearable or to assist in handling the normal stresses of daily living. It may be that you know students who seem to use these devices to the extent that they seem almost out of touch with reality. This is, however, no sign that they are ready for counseling, or that you have the right or obligation to get involved. The overuse of defense mechanisms is symptomatic of maladjustment. A good rule of thumb would seem to be that *counseling is indicated when defense mechanisms begin to break down.* When the student can no longer convince herself that her behavior is excusable or understandable, she is probably ready to accept help. As a counselor, your most effective role may be in helping the student rebuild defenses so that she can once again live with herself with some degree of emotional comfort.

Another potential problem may be the result of the behavior of the faculty member during the counseling session. This refers particularly to the areas of *timing, pacing, tone of voice,* and *nonverbal communication.* Timing refers to the sixth sense or intuitive feeling developed by experienced counselors that enables them to know the appropriate moment to introduce something into the counseling session, such as threatening material, active direction by the counselor or specific recommendations for action. At the right time in a counseling relationship the counselor may direct, initiate, diagnose, advise, and have the student understand and accept. Poor timing may result in a broken relationship as the student is frightened away.

Pacing refers to the speed with which a counselor talks. Students may come in highly agitated and excited, to the extent that they talk extremely rapidly. The faculty member can help to restore the student gradually to a more normal pattern by continuing to talk in a normal manner, calm and reasonably slow. This also allows both the faculty member and the student to listen more, to absorb what is being said, and to think a little more clearly. The tone of voice is equally important because it serves to convey to the student an air of calmness, confidence, and security—the faculty member is not upset and excited, the student begins to feel that she can get help here.

The whole area of nonverbal communication is frequently overlooked. We need to be much more aware of the student's nonverbal messages to us which are conveyed particularly through her eyes, mouth, hands, and general body posture. These signals can tell us a great deal about the feelings of the student such as tension, anger, withdrawal. We also need to develop a much greater awareness of our own nonverbal signals which may convey incorrect messages to the student, such as anger, impatience, disinterest. A good way for a faculty member to check out her own nonverbal behavior is for her to ask her colleagues or her students for regular feedback about the messages she seems to be sending and they are receiving.

The student who is to be counseled should be the center of the counseling process, and the faculty member providing counseling should be constantly sensitive to her. Basic to success in counseling is an understanding of the student's concept of herself, her readiness and freedom for action, her inner conflicts and suppressed desires, her unwarranted feelings of fear and guilt, her inner springs of behavior—in short, why she behaves as she does. Her physical condition and her concept of the counselor's role are also of paramount importance.

The student is seeking self-realization, self-actualization, and self-fulfillment; she is hoping to make her life more complete and satisfying. She has the capacity within herself to do this, although at times she may need assistance. Confucius embodied this principle in his saying, "Remember that thou art man and frail and likely to fall; but if thou fall, remember thou art man and have it within thyself to get up." Conditions giving rise to any given kind of human development are infinitely complex. Hereditary nervous instability, mental retardation, disease and other physical conditions, family pressures, cultural and racial background, the influence of friends, "the neurotic personality of our times," and various inner conflicts may all be involved in any individual's adjustment. None of these factors acts singly. Even symptoms serve a purpose. They indicate the existence of a problem, and show how the student is attempting to solve it. They also frequently act as a safety valve; they sometimes prevent something worse from happening. For some students, their behavior serves as a bright red warning flag signalling loudly and clearly, "I need help."

None of the foregoing suggests that you should be diagnosing personality disorders. It does suggest, however, that as nurse educators we cannot avoid making necessary judgments about behavior, and that as nursing educators we have at least minimal contact with symptoms of personality breakdown and psychological stress.

# Chapter 5

# *Special Concerns of the Nursing Student*

The previous chapters have provided a basis for guidance and counseling services in schools of nursing. We have dealt with counseling principles and techniques, and the general concerns of the college student. The purpose of this chapter will be to examine some specialized concerns that are highly prevalent among nursing students and require teaching and information dissemination or counseling intervention and assistance.

## INDIVIDUALITY AND THE ROLE OF THE NURSE

Recent trends in the development of most helping professions include the acceptance of the humanistic aspect of the individual without the subversion or rejection of human feelings and emotions. For example, some nursing educators used to argue that an impersonal, objective, professional attitude must be maintained in order to deal competently with the needs of the patient. Educators felt that a student without such defenses would be unable to provide adequate care for the patient. They further felt that the humanistic approach to the treatment situation could seriously jeopardize the patient's welfare. Today it has become a matter of deep concern to nursing educators as to how the young student learns to handle the feelings aroused in her as she deals with the needs of the patient. How does she manage those feelings aroused by a relationship which is often more intimate and trying than any found outside of nursing?

Female students may show concern for being a woman first and a nurse second. Male nursing students may show concern as to whether the role of a nurse will add to or detract from the stereotyped role of the male in our society. The traditional expectation of the nursing role was one of impersonal competence and efficiency with the added qualities of purity, piety, and perseverance. The nurse was expected to refrain from involvement in situations in which her feelings would be expressed in public. In fact, in many instances her personal life was not hers to govern and live; the school of nursing or the hospital saw to it that the student had a clear knowledge and understanding of what was and was not proper nurse behavior. These traditional expectations may occasionally be found today among members of the "old guard," and may cause negative reactions on the part of nursing students who represent the new generation. In other words, how does a student nurse reconcile her personal feelings toward herself and her patients with the professional role she is expected to fill?

## SEXUALITY AND NURSING

Some authorities in nursing education and professional nursing indicate that the nurse who has denied her human aspect runs a high risk in any interpersonal relationship, ranging from patient care to marriage. It would appear from the foregoing that nursing educators must make themselves available to students who need basic information or counseling assistance in working through their feelings about sex and sexuality, especially in relation to patient care. Strong restrictive social conditioning of the human individual, erotically relevant fantasies at a given stage of sexual development, and the link between sexual pleasure and reproduction may be bases for individual and group discussion and counseling (Stephens, 1970). In the human being the sexual relationship is optional, and can vary along an entire spectrum from pleasure sensations totally devoid of reproductive possibility to the indulgence in heterosexual intercourse solely for the purpose of begetting a child. It may be necessary to help students contend with an apparent sexual revolution manifested by an increased acknowledgment by the diverse segments of Western society that a mindless conformity to external criteria of acceptable or permissible sexual activity, whether imposed by the state, church, family or the self in the form of internalized restrictions, is not necessary or desirable for either the individual or society. Stephens indicates that ultimately the revolution in sexual mores and practice is an expression of individual demands for sexual determination. One's sexual activity can and should be a matter of conscious personal choice based on one's own needs and desires. Counseling can help students arrive at this point, able to make rational decisions for themselves based on knowledge and acceptance of self.

The student also needs an opportunity to gain an understanding of the role her sex will play in the profession she has chosen. For example, discriminatory practices based on the sex of the nurse must be considered. Cleland (1971) indicates that too often the nurse allows male domination of her profession. This domination may manifest itself in many ways, but most characteristically in salaries and the range of authority and administration. In fact, sex discrimination may increase through the increasing number of male nurses who are seeking supervisory, teaching, and administrative jobs within nursing. It is also fostered through the male-dominated ranks of physicians, and the "hero worship" in which the nurse looks up to the man as the leader.

## SEX EDUCATION

To what extent is sex education a responsibility of the school of nursing? What role should the nursing educator play in dealing with students who may be encountering a sexual or reproductive crisis? Does the nursing educator advise and counsel the student according to the student's values or according to the values and the dictates of the institution? Does the nursing faculty take the time to understand fully the impact of the crisis on the student? Can the student be provided counseling which will help her make her own choice? Depending on the answers to these questions will be the student's attitude toward nursing care for patients in similar situations.

On the basis of available evidence it would seem that nursing students need sex education for themselves, and to equip them to deal with patients' problems in the sexual and reproductive areas. It would seem logical and desirable for schools of nursing to take on this role. Thus the authors feel quite strongly that courses in Human Sexuality should be built in as part of the curriculum of every school of nursing.

Advances in birth control techniques have allowed almost complete freedom from the fear of pregnancy. With this reduction in fear has come a greater freedom in the attitudes toward premarital and extramarital sex. At least to some extent, it would seem to be the school of nursing's responsibility to help each student learn to accept this freedom in a responsible fashion. Single working women, of whom the nurse may be one, have the highest rate of illegitimate births next to teenagers, in spite of birth control. Acceptance of sexual freedom without guilt and feelings of loss of personal worth and reprisal on the part of the single working nurse may require expert advice and counsel.

It is not uncommon to find in any segment of our population homosexuality as a means of satisfying sexual identification and needs. A great fear among students may be attributed to their suspicions that they are homosexual because they have strong positive feelings toward someone of the same sex. Students watch for manifestations of latent homosexuality in examining their own feelings and relationships with others. Nursing educators are presented a task of serious proportions in establishing an atmosphere in which these kinds of concerns can be aired openly with feelings of trust and confidentiality. This task is at least partially created by the large number of single women in the schools and profession of nursing. Here again, counseling on an individual and group basis, and sex education classes may be useful in assisting students to handle these concerns.

## MEN IN NURSING

The dominant image presently being emphasized for male nurses is that nursing is and can become more of a masculine occupation. Fosberg (1969) describes his experiences as a nurse involved in the air evacuation of Vietnam military personnel. The emphasis of the article was that in war areas and in other critical situations, men were better able to serve and, more importantly, were expected to serve better than their female counterparts. Without debating the merits of the article, the image presented is one of high risk taking, of heroic dedication, and very masculine. In contrast, Aldag and Cristensen (1967) found that the personality profile of male nursing students, as measured by the MMPI, was more similar to that of female nursing students than the profiles of male or female junior college students. The MF scale analysis indicated that male and female nursing students are more feminine than male or female junior college students. This finding is not particularly surprising since nursing fills a mothering or nurturant role. Men can fill this mothering or nurturant role just as women can fill a father role when they become physicians. The underlying character structure of nursing students in the Aldag and Cristensen study more often included the passive-dependent and less often the aggressive, rebellious traits when compared with male and female junior college students. Here again, students may need counseling if these feelings interfere with their performance or their personal comfort.

Other evidences of sensitivity to the enrollment of men into schools of nursing can sometimes be found in the clinical training areas. It should be stressed that this problem is receiving growing recognition and is beginning to be dealt with by nursing educators. Nevertheless both students and faculty members need to develop a greater awareness in this area. For example, some nursing educators attempt to minimize the impact of male students' presence in obstetrics and gynecology by providing minimal training to them in these particular areas. There appears to be differential concern here in that male students face greater acceptance in obstetrics than in gynecology wards by the nursing staff. Most nursing staffs in gynecology indicate that the nature of the treatment necessary would make female patients feel uncomfortable if male students were present.

It appears, however, that little research has been done to investigate the degree to which service on a gynecology unit for male nurses would be a detriment to the patient. No efforts to identify the areas of negative impact and the degree of impact have been reported in the research literature. This is not too surprising, for it would be difficult to reconcile such findings with the fact that most women have male physicians. It would seem that we may be dealing more with the expectations and attitudes of society, the hospital, and the staff in anticipating problems in this area. Some nursing educators claim that they have no problems in that they allow complete access to all training services for all students, provided that for the student's protection a female nurse goes with the male student to the obstetric-gynecology area or is there to supervise. Interestingly enough, the opposite does not hold true in these schools; i.e. there is no provision for a male nurse to go with a female nurse to the genitourinary unit. These training situations may indicate the degree of comfort in cross-sex working and interpersonal relationships for the nursing faculty.

Specialization within nursing for male nurses, as indicated by female nursing educators, would be particularly available in nonbedside nursing such as anesthesia, administration, supervision, education, and psychiatric nursing. Although there may be some concern for male nurses about maintenance of a masculine image, the unfortunate preference of some female nurses for men to take on the positions of leadership may, in time, significantly alter the profession from one of being predominantly female to one of equal numbers of men and women under male leadership. Cleland (1971) is critical of the female leadership within nursing which seems to adhere to the concept of male superiority. She indicates that the situation described above is a good indication of the need to dictate equality for female nurses through female leadership.

Every effort should be made to orient the student to treating patients of the opposite sex. The fact that both sexes are present in the same student body could result in some highly relevant and meaningful group discussion, interaction, and role playing. An attitude of openness on the part of both faculty and students will provide a basis for individual and group exploration of the meaning of sex and sexuality for themselves and for the patients they are to serve. The students need help in overcoming self-consciousness and temerity in accepting sexual identity and the physical aspects of the body. One cannot assume that "knowing the physiology of how babies are made" is all that a nurse needs to know about sex. Awkwardness in dealing with a sexually awkward problem could result in a situation in which the nurse is ineffective and the patient suffers.

Abortion, acceptance of loss, change of body image, and death and dying require further self-examination by the student nurse. Younger students may suffer the greater shock, and the need for assistance in acceptance and adjustment. For example, many articles written by nurses and by nursing students who find themselves terminally ill or caring for terminally ill patients dramatize the need for nursing faculty and student nurses to examine carefully their attitudes, expectations, perceptions, and convictions in these matters.

## ABORTION

In a study by Brown et al. (1971), nurses responded to a question about abortion in a manner similar to that of female physicians. Both groups favored abortion less than male physicians under all circumstances except by decision of a health board. Nurses are not usually asked to serve on such boards. The situation may give some good indications of areas for discussion about involvement and decision making and the sharing of responsibility for the total care of the patient by nursing staff. It appears that nursing staffs are comfortable to have others decide what to do, what risks are to be taken, and when to intervene with the idea of prevention. Younger female university hospital nurses were more likely to condone abortion. Variation was present among specialty groups. Nurses on the premature care centers were more in favor of abortion for all reasons than were nurses in the delivery and postpartum units, nursery, and pediatric services. There was a gradient of increasing support from single to married to widowed to separated-divorced nurses for abortion for medical and economic-social reasons. There were strong associations of marital status with attitudes toward abortion.

Fonseca (1968) indicates that nurses must examine their personal definitions of nursing before they can accept the responsibilities of professional care in the management of unwanted pregnancy. Some may view induced abortion as a serious public health problem, while others would view it as a means of alleviating a serious public health problem. Fonseca argues that "if a nurse in good conscience cannot accept any part in the nursing care of women before, during or after an induced abortion, her negation of responsibility will affect her nursing care in all facets of her professional life."

An example of this conflict can be seen in the statement released by the Massachusetts Nurses Association in July, 1971, which followed the statement of the California State Nurses Association in December, 1970. The MNA policy states: "Unless the patient's life is in jeopardy, professional nurses shall not be required to participate in therapeutic abortions, tubal ligations, vasectomies or other practices which may be in conflict with their ethical or religious beliefs." On the other hand, the MNA statement affirms that "the professional nurses shall not discourage, dissuade or attempt to dissuade by affirmative action or silence, any patient from seeking or receiving reasonable treatment where objection to such treatment arises because of the ethical or religious beliefs of the nurse."

Nurses, as a group, tend to reflect societal norms in terms of moral codes, mores, ethics, and attitudes. The nurse, perhaps inappropriately, will judge patients by these standards. Labelling the patient as "good" or "bad" can be attributed to how deviant from the standard norms are the adapted behaviors of the patient. Thus it may be that those who require public assistance are "bad" or "ignorant," since they represent a lower socioeconomic group which differs from the norms. It is more likely for women in ward situations to be labelled "bad," and the women in private rooms to be considered "good" or "better." Does the nurse, and should she, judge the morality of the patient, or account for differences in patients' ability to cope with their situations? How will nurse judgments of morality, and the accounting for coping behaviors, affect the kind and quality of nursing care in the treatment of induced abortion? Research indicates that individuals respond and behave in ways authorities (nurses) expect them to behave. Nurse perceptions due to biased expectations may lead to self-fulfilling prophecies, and subsequent mismanagement of patient care.

Student nurses are caught up in the same ambivalent feelings as graduate nurses. The student nurse's image of her role as nurse and as woman may be critically affected by prior growth experiences, nursing education practices, and modeling of significant others. Caring for patients who deviate in any way from the student's expectations can arouse difficulties in providing meaningful patient care. Counseling on an individual or group basis is in order to assist students in overcoming confrontation with other people's standards and norms, and to help them put aside their own value system in order to provide good nursing care.

## ACCEPTANCE OF LOSS

Nursing students may experience extreme negative reactions to patients suffering loss of identification, body parts or function. The treatment of such a patient will depend significantly upon the degree to which the student has viewed the potential or actual loss of her own body parts or function. Does the student understand the concept of loss in relationship to the total individual? Loss of body parts or function may or may not mean loss of identity as a person of worth. For some students, working with a patient who is undergoing the grief and mourning of loss will arouse feelings of inadequacy, guilt, and perhaps a sense of relief that it is the patient's loss and not the student's. Students may need help in resolving these ambivalent feelings. Wright (1960) indicates that professionals who are working with patients suffering loss need to understand the impact of loss on the self, self-identification, and the ability to adjust and to cope with acceptance. Students will need help through individual and group counseling in working with patients who fight the loss, and who treat themselves as useless and, for all intents and purposes, dead. Students also need help in understanding that, for some patients, the loss of a diseased part of the body is welcomed and accepted. In other words, they must learn that no two individuals will necessarily react the same way to the same situation.

## THE NURSING STUDENT AND THE DYING PATIENT

The nursing educator confronted with the task of preparing her students to meet the complex needs of the terminal patient is indeed involved in a multifaceted dilemma. The very nature of her educational role is to direct her students through the theoretical and practical measures by which the future nurse will emerge as a person strongly oriented toward life, its beginning, its health, and its longevity. Paradoxically, this intense orientation toward the preservation of human life can be one of the greatest obstacles to the future nurse's role as one who must, on one hand, intimately assist her patients to die with dignity and acceptance and, at the same time, meet the expectations of medical staff and the family of the terminal patient. The reader's attention is called to an exemplary in-depth analysis of the role of the student nurse as she meets the needs of the terminal patient (Quint, 1967).

The perceptions of the nursing educator in her role as educating about death arise from several sources. She is the principal resource for the student nurse in the matters of death and dying. As such, she functions out of a multiplicity of her own attitudes and expectations regarding the terminal patient, those of the physicians with whom she has worked, those of the patients themselves, and, most important, those of the neophyte nurses who as yet are ambivalent in their perceptions of death—their own, and those to whom they will minister in their clinical responsibilities. Two important factors should then be considered. How do the living feel about dying, and how do the dying feel about death?

If one were to assume that the experienced nurse's attitude and feelings toward death are akin to those of physicians, the picture would indeed be bleak. Paul S. Rhoads, reporting at the 1964 AMA Meeting, states that his research of a liberal sampling of physician attitudes toward the terminal patient resulted in a conclusion that some 70 per cent of these physicians did not inform their patients that they were facing terminal illness (Rhoads, 1964). If this is the prevailing attitude of physicians, what, then, can be expected of the nurse who must work within the limitations set forth by the physicians under and with whom she must work daily?

The answer to this question is graphically given by Bowers et al. (1964) as they portray the behavioral masks worn by physicians and nurses in their approach to the terminal patient. These authors are really describing denial behaviors resorted to by medical personnel, which is one of the principal barriers to the patient's accepting, in a healthy manner, his imminent death. The first "mask" is the use of professional language, whereby the physician or nurse knows what he or she is saying, but is quite sure that the words have little or no meaning for the patient. Responses to the oft-repeated question by patients, when inquiring about their illness, such as, "Oh, you have a glioblastoma," or, "We've discovered that you have Burkitt's lymphoma," really tell most patients nothing, but they do assuage the guilt of the physician or nurse and assure him or her of a pseudo-honesty that he or she has responded to the patient's inquiry.

Another "mask" impeding a person-to-person relationship with the patient is that of cynicism. This particular response to the terminal patient can be acquired early in the professional preparation of a nurse, as well as a physician. It is a defense against the reality of death that is met often in surgery and the performance of autopsies. The student nurse will first learn this defense from the verbalized expressions of the surgeon when, in the process of an exploratory laparotomy, the surgeon discovers the irreversible metastasis of a well developed carcinoma and, upon his discovery, remarks, "Close him up; he's had his last steak," or some such jocular remark. Such cynicism begets in the mind of the assisting student nurse not only a sense of hopelessness, but also of helplessness, and jocular cynicism can rapidly displace these bad feelings.

One of the most common "masks" or defenses against the reality of death is the "mask of materiality." Medical instrumentation is used to divert the patient's direct inquiry about his condition or his silent plea for clarification. The oral thermometer literally shuts off verbal communication between patient and nurse; the earpieces reaching down to the blood pressure cuff render the nurse "legitimately deaf" to inquiry.

Another "mask" found to be an effective defense is that of impersonality. In this the nurse refers to the patient as "the pneumonectomy in 319" or "the CVA in 420." These references to the terminal patient render him less and less personal and more and more "a case."

"Ritualized action," which is really impersonal ritualized interaction, also spares the nurse feelings of inadequacy and threat. It would seem that many of the traditional person-to-person nurse-patient interactions have decreased in frequency through the services of the aides who are more and more assuming the functions of taking blood pressures and temperatures, heretofore functions of the registered nurse. Probably the most frequent interaction between patient and nurse is to be found in the administration of medications. Even this opportunity for the patient to verbalize his needs is limited when the patient is handed the oral medications and a glass of water, the ingestion of both allowing him little chance to discuss his condition or express fears and needs. Many patients have related their reluctance, and even guilt, at talking to the nurse simply because they see the quantity of drugs on her tray which tell them that the nurse is busy and must get to the next patient.

Hospitals, as institutions, must function with some degrees and kinds of routines. These routines can assist the nurse in restricting her interaction with the terminal patient. Interruptions by housekeeping staff, the paper boy entering the room unannounced, the visiting hours and the presence of visitors—all can effectively limit the opportunities for nurse-patient interaction as a personal exploration by the nurse about how the patient feels about his imminent death. All the above-described nurse-to-patient avoidance behaviors and "masks" graphically portray the reality that the nurse is literally afraid of the terminal patient.

The student nurse may also be called upon to cope with the feelings of the family of the terminal patient. The student's education about death, previous to her formal nursing education, will have been grossly lacking in the fundamentals of death and bereavement. Death education as a part of family life education has little to offer the current nursing student, according to the most recent research (Somerville, 1971). Somerville states, "It has been said that death and sex are the two subjects parents find most difficult to talk about with their children." She goes on to describe the absence of this form of education in the elementary, secondary, and college years of education in America. Thus the nursing educator is faced with the problem of helping the student to explore and develop not only her own understanding and feelings about death, but also those of the families of the terminally ill patient so that all three—patient, family, and nurse—can approach imminent death in as positive and healthy a manner as possible. Herman Feifel (1959), writing about attitudes toward death, tells us that "a review of the psychiatric and psychological literature highlights the lack of any systematic endeavors to bring this area into the domain of controlled investigation."

Thus we can come to a number of conclusions about how the living feel about the dying. The behaviors of medical and nursing personnel and the virtual absence of formal educational resources for the general population point to a picture of fear among all, and specifically a fear of being a part of the dying patient's reality. Physicians, nurses, and patient's families will go to rather extreme measures to avoid what the patient appears to need most—open communications and the opportunity to talk about his death (Ross, 1969). This is the primary reason why we feel so strongly the need for individual and group counseling with student nurses on this subject.

How do the dying feel about death? The response to this question can provide vastly important insights for the student nurse in the care of the terminally ill.

Doctor Elizabeth Kubler-Ross (1969) presents an excellent portrayal of the stages of emotional adjustment to the awareness of imminent death. The following explanation should give the reader an overview of the intensity and duration of these stages.

Initial shock is highly intense, but brief in duration. This reaction is one of silent numbness. Its cessation is usually followed by passive or active denial, a behavior that rises and ebbs during the following stages of anger, bargaining, and preparatory grief and depression, and hopefully culminates in the acceptance stage. It can begin as passive in the sense that the patient does not take action on it, but wonders about the possibilities that the diagnosis is inaccurate, that a mistake has been made in the laboratory or that someone has interpreted the wrong x-rays. Concomitant with this form of denial can be strong feelings of anger that he or she should have been so badly victimized by the physician's error. The feelings then shift from passive denial, often verbalized as "This can't be," to the more agitated kinds of active denial whereby the patient may persist in saying to himself and others, "Not only is it true that I can't be dying, but I am not dying." This avoidance fantasy often motivates the patient to seek out a multiplicity of physicians and diagnostic procedures to confirm the error of the original terminal diagnosis and reinforce his conviction that he is, in fact, not dying. This patient will seek to shift discussion about death to trite matters, will appear cheerful, and even at times project an air of indifference about his condition. Ross (1969) emphasizes the positive and necessary value of denial for the patient at this stage. "What I am trying to emphasize is that the need for denial exists in every patient at times, at the very beginning of illness more so than at the end of life. Later on the need comes and goes, and the sensitive and perceptive listener will acknowledge this and allow the patient his defenses without making him aware of the contradictions."

It is relevant here to call attention to the opportunities available through the behaviors of the terminally ill for valuable insights into many problem-coping situations for all people and most especially hospital personnel. The dying patient can be a highly effective teacher for all of us in attaining appropriate coping behaviors, since we are often faced with stress and conflict situations. Virginia Barckley (1964) points out that one of the most effective lessons to be learned from the dying is that "death is not defeat," and this realization should have the highest priority on the student nurse's initial awareness of and approach to the terminal patient.

Subsequent to initial shock and denial, the terminal patient, finally having assessed his imminent death, will ask himself, "If it is true that I am dying, why me?" The student nurse should anticipate that the patient will become angry, envious of the living, and that he will displace or project his anger to his family and hospital personnel. Terminal patients at this stage will reflect this anger in caustic remarks about the hospital and its staff, become quite uncooperative in responding to treatment, highly critical of food, and hostile to the persons rendering these services. Nursing personnel who are responding to this anger with anger and impatience should be asked whether they too would not react in like manner if they were told that their world were to end tomorrow. The terminal patient often expresses a sense of urgency to get as much accomplished as possible during whatever life space is to be allotted to him (Brainard, 1971). Many hospital procedures call for just the opposite. The nurse frequently, verbally or nonverbally, is telling the patient to "be inactive" as she inserts the intravenous needle or prepares the patient for such procedures as transfusions, electrocardiograms, temperature and blood pressure recordings, replacement of surgical dressings, and so many other functions that call for physical passivity on the part of the patient. This conflict—the patient's need to be active and the nurse's need that he be inactive—can trigger frustrations on the part of both and reinforce anger, indeed prolong it. It is during this stage that families, friends, and hospital personnel resolutely seek means to avoid interaction with the patient. Were they to realize that this anger is rational and justifiable, given the patient's fears and feelings, perhaps their reactions to the patient would change from rejection to a response to a plea for help and concern.

The third stage in the sequence of the death process has been called "bargaining" (Ross, 1969), and is described well by Brauer (1960) as he perceives the patient at this stage. This stage may be viewed as the pseudo-hope response behavior of the terminal patient. During this period the patient seeks to postpone his death through such means as offering himself as a living subject for cancer research with some newly discovered chemotherapy, asking for further diagnostic tests and consultations, even seeking out medical quacks selling their "cures" and cure-alls. Some patients will make a silent pact with God that, in return for an extension of life, they will return to a life of outstanding virtue.

It seems appropriate at this stage to offer some observations on "hope" in the spectrum of the terminal patient's behaviors and expectations. The literature in this area presents a rather firm consensus that at no time should all hope be stricken from the patient's realm of realization and fantasy. Whether the patient's hope be therapeutic or antagonistically unrealistic is a product of several factors. The method of disclosure will be of paramount importance. The physician, who holds principal responsibility for disclosure, may be blunt or subtle. If Rhoads is correct in his findings, direct or indirect disclosure more often than not will not take place through the physician. Thus the patient will be left in a state of doubt, and hope for him becomes a conflict rather than an adjunct to accepting his situation.

Verwoerdt and Wilson (1967) tell us that the essential issue is not "whether the patient should be told, but rather, how he should be told." "Hope is the anticipation of good prospects in the future," Elmore and Verwoerdt (1967) tell us. It may be hypothesized that either extreme—blunt disclosure or no disclosure—will heighten and prolong the patient's shock, denial, anger, bargaining, and depression and thereby reduce his accepting in a positive manner his imminent death. The patient's past history of using realistic hope as a coping mechanism will be another factor determining his response to disclosure or self-awareness of approaching death, and thus his degree of realistic hope. Ultimately the patient, and all concerned with him, will ask themselves, "What basis is there for hope?"

The response to this is, of course, determined by the nature and extent of the terminal disease. Cardiac and renal dysfunctional patients have certainly been granted more optimism of late through recent progress in surgical and transplant procedures. The National Cancer Institute, through Doctor Carl G. Baker (1971), informs us that seven forms of cancer, accounting for 15 per cent of all known forms of cancer, are currently responding to chemotherapy. The same source points to the important discoveries about the properties and functions of RNA and especially DNA molecules and relation to cancer origin and cure as presenting a more optimistic therapeutic picture. The nurse can provide realistic kinds of hope for the terminal patient by making known to him this progress in science. This can be done only if the nurse seeks skills in departing from the mask of professional language, interpreting the current state of medical resources for his illness in terms understandable and interesting to the patient. This approach has been found to be most effective when responding to the patient's questions relating to prognosis and regression. It also enhances the patient's progress through the bargaining stage of his emotional reaction to impending death. It should be noted here that some patients may use denial right to the point of death. Also, the nurse is bound by the decisions of the physician; if she feels that the patient wants to know, she must get the physician to agree.

The fourth stage in the dying process described by Ross is that of depression and preparatory grief. Shock, numbness, denial, and anger have abated significantly. Some degrees of bargaining may remain, but one sees the patient as perceiving himself as lost. In many cases he has incurred physical loss through surgery, financial loss through health expenses, great social alienation through the avoidance behaviors of family and hospital personnel, and eventually a loss of will to live. This depression is further reinforced by impending loss of a different kind. As Ross (1969) tells us, this calls for a different understanding and approach by those meeting the needs of the dying patient. She refers to initial depression as reactive and its culmination being preparatory depression. She sees the former as best responded to with frequent and concrete depression-alleviating behaviors by family and hospital personnel, and the latter as best alleviated by allowing the patient to be depressed, the depression being a tool to prepare for acceptance.

Thus response to reactive depression would take the forms of encouragement and reassurances, while the latter depression would allow the patient more time to be alone with his thoughts, a minimum of fictitious encouragements, and a reduction of interfering kinds of behaviors by family and staff, such as extended and frequent visits and prolongation of unnecessary treatments. The patient would seem to need this time to be introspective, to plan his next decisions, and to develop acceptance of imminent death. Critical to this stage is allowing the patient to determine his environment, decisions about future treatments, and the acceptance of his family and staff that he is dying. Paradoxically, it too often happens that family and hospital personnel, in their frustrations, almost beseige the patient with demands reflecting their professional and cultural expectations, but grossly contrary to his needs at this stage. The nurse should not have to experience guilt by reducing interaction with the patient in this stage; it may be his preference that interaction be reduced so that he can think and prepare and finally accept his situation. Often, however, nurses leave the patient alone because of their need rather than his.

Should the patient have progressed through the first four stages, he will enter that phase that Ross calls "acceptance." She warns us that "acceptance is not necessarily a happy state of affairs, it is a period of time almost devoid of feelings." The patient wants our physical presence, but with little verbal communication, and that according to what he wants to express, not what we want to tell him. Communication among patient, family, and hospital personnel will be tacit or explicit, frequent or rare, verbal or nonverbal, according to the needs of the patient at this stage. The nurse should be especially aware of what the patient is saying nonverbally during this time if she is to facilitate his progress through acceptance.

The final stage of death, decathexis, is a process of detachment from the environment and the significant others in the patient's life. It is characterized by frequent sleeping spells, almost total disinterest in treatment procedures, and a desire to be left alone with the exception of the presence of a member of the family who is most aware of the death process and its concomitant needs. It is brief and in a way mirrors the first few days of an infant's life, mostly sleep interspersed with periodic arousal to limited awareness of what is going on around him. This is not a process of rejection, and it is vitally important that the nurse convey this message to the family and more importantly realize it herself lest she perceive herself as being rejected after a long period of being a meaningful person in that patient's life. It is a time when the needs of the family rather than those of the patient should take priority in the nurse's role. It is the family now that needs reassuring that they have done all they could possibly do, and that they have done it well. The nurse should clarify to the family that this final detachment stage is a normal process, highly beneficial to the patient, and thank them for whatever contributions the family has made to the patient in his dying situation. The nurse should take pride in her contribution to the patient, overcoming her own fears, masks, impatience, and anger, and, most important, her acceptance of the realities of death. This may be the point at which the nurse herself needs counseling assistance to help her handle her own feelings.

In summary, the role of the nursing educator is seen as essentially initiating and developing attitudes about death. These attitudes, or habitual reactions, must come from within the mind and feelings of the educator if she is to function effectively as a facilitator or change agent in responding to the needs of her students in this realm of nursing care. The mere integration of new ideas about death will not be enough. Her nonverbalized feelings, both in the classroom and during clinical supervision, will be the most effective and convincing methodology for initiating and developing healthy attitudes in her students toward the terminal patient.

Caring for a terminally ill patient may arouse strong feelings which the student nurse may find difficult to control. This situation has its greatest impact when there has been a close relationship between the patient and the nurse. Nursing students should be prepared for the many different ways people prepare for death or deny its inevitability. The fact that patients prepare for death in unexpected ways should be made known to the student. In many instances the patient finds it easier to accept his death than does the student nurse. Students need to understand that patients, regardless of the nursing intervention, will work through the process of dying in their own way. There is enough evidence of this in the studies reported by Ross (1969). A more critical issue is the management of death and dying by the student. How does the student prepare herself for treating the dying patient? Will this be the first experience for the student in being near someone who is dying? Has the student avoided thinking about death and its significance? In contrast, how does the student manage thoughts about life and the living? Students need time and assistance to consider these kinds of questions, and their role as a nurse in the postponement of death.

Brown et al. (1971) indicate in their study that nurses show a higher percentage of affirmative responses for euthanasia. Positive euthanasia, when steps are taken by the treatment team (if they had the legal right to do so from a patient, and the recommendation from a health board which had legal sanction), could alleviate prolonged, needless suffering. The more experienced the nurse was in dealing with death and separation in her personal and professional life, the more she favored positive euthanasia. The study, however, in no way prepares one in how to interact with a patient who is faced with death and knows it. Some students really take issue with the whole concept of euthanasia, since they see themselves as able to prolong life rather than to help end it. They must be helped to work through the question as to whether the nurse has the right to intervene either way. Can the student respond to the patient in a warm, concerned manner, or is she too involved with her own feelings? Unless death is sudden, will the student be able to share the fears, anxieties, denial, pleading, and withdrawal of the patient? Will the student have enough inner resources to provide a supportive hand to the patient as she dies?

The student must also become aware that people may be encountered who steadfastly refuse medical treatment because of religious beliefs, although the incidence of such cases appears to be minimal. The faith most of us have in the omniscience of medicine and our personal belief in the value of a human life can lead us, as well as the student, to the denial of the right of the patient and his family to refuse treatment. Nursing educators should be able to deal immediately and directly with evidences of intolerance or derogation of the patient's values and beliefs. The desire to help may be so strong that the student is blinded to the motives for her actions. Again, counseling is needed in this area.

The remaining family members may also require support from the nurse. Will she be able to give it? Will she be of any help to the family in its struggle to move through the various stages of the dying process to ultimate acceptance? Will the nurse be of assistance and support as the family deals with the dying family member? Separation and the acceptance of loss may cause severe trauma among the remaining family members. Children especially may need expert help in overcoming the separation from significant adults, and the nurse has a vital role here. Is it within the realm of the nursing role to act as a parent or significant other in the life of a very small patient? We would hope that the nurse will be able to respond to the demands for security, comfort, and love made by a very small patient. This will not happen unless she has been helped, while still a student, to prepare herself for this role.

## THE CULTURALLY DIFFERENT STUDENT

Nursing educators today are faced with the ever-increasing challenge of providing relevant educational and professional opportunities for the culturally different student. This includes the provision of meaningful advising and counseling when necessary. Although the following discussion is primarily concerned with the black student, the concerns expressed apply equally to the educational and vocational needs of other minority group students.

Cultural disadvantage is not a diagnosis of disability, but a set of unique, multiple, interacting symptoms. No single term adequately identifies the condition. Disadvantage involves social, educational, economic, and cultural deprivation, and may be relative or absolute. Its consequences are serious for the nursing educator, student, and the vast potential patient population. Disadvantage, as a symptom, exists to a greater degree among blacks, Puerto Ricans, Chicanos, and American Indians than for the majority of white Americans.

Some common psychological attributes arise from the role and place of the disadvantaged in society: a different performance on educational, psychological, and other behavioral tasks; a different language and verbal expression which pose subtle difficulties in communication and concurrent learning; pervasive attitudes which appear to be self-defeating; a higher incidence of social maladaptive behavior, including passivity, crime, and emotional disturbance. Because of unmet physical needs, a particularly strong need for security may arise which negates their ability to work toward long-term goals. Preferences for short-term goals with tangible pleasures develop. For example, the disadvantaged nursing student more often is found in LPN or AD programs because of their shorter training periods.

In spite of these shortcomings, the disadvantaged appear to aspire to better things. Their efforts to improve their status through educational and vocational attainment are often influenced by many kinds of subtle self-defeating and conflicting behaviors. From a psychological point of view, the disadvantaged, minority group student may have poor examples or "role models" in their parents or significant others who have been unable to develop or demonstrate effective coping behaviors. In addition, she may have few if any role models in nursing leadership positions.

Counseling and guidance strategies that are currently applied to the disadvantaged are based primarily on principles and theory taken from the psychology and education of the nondisadvantaged. Thus important counseling theories have serious limitations when applied to work with the disadvantaged. If counseling is to be used with the disadvantaged student, considerable modification in theory and goals may be needed. Social and cultural differences may place a counselor in the hazardous position of inappropriately judging the student nurse as unable to accommodate significant academic or personal change. One might reasonably anticipate difficulty in establishing a trusting relationship. The counselor who emphasizes self-actualization or any other theoretical approach to counseling may invite student rejection of counseling. Typical educational, psychological, and vocational testing may place the student in an unfair, dependent, subordinate position because of culturally biased tests. This point will be discussed further in Chapter 11.

Counselors and faculty members should be sensitive to the impact of the environment from which the disadvantaged student comes. They should be able to recognize and to cope with subtle, cultural maskings of hostility, anxiety, and fear of failure. Most importantly, they should be able to deal with individual motivational differences and sensitivities and their own feelings and frame of reference.

Maximizing the development of relevant learning approaches and job skills is necessary in order to achieve equality of professional preparation and opportunity for practice for the culturally different student. For example, some writers claim that the black student shows differential learning sets and abilities (Jensen, 1964). It may be that the black student shows an equal ability with whites in learning associative tasks, but displays a deficit in abstract tasks. If this is true, then the emphasis for learning could be the conversion of abstract learning tasks into associative tasks. In addition, the recruitment of culturally different students should take this into consideration.

Henke (1971) describes a tutorial advancing program (TAP) which involved counseling, financial assistance, and the provision of remedial services in reading, arithmetic, and grammar for culturally different students whose grade point averages were too low for them to be considered for acceptance into nursing school. These services are needed because of the inequality of students' high school education. The goal was to increase educational attainment and readiness for admission to regular nursing educational programs. Results indicate a success ratio of 50 per cent; i.e. four out of eight made it. The study showed that one-to-one relationships were vital to successful performance. Group discussions, living together, and experience in a hospital with patients

proved to be the factors preferred by the students. Organized to-
getherness and sightseeing enculturation proved to be negative factors
for the students. The study suggests that by altering an orientation to
nursing and nursing academics, otherwise marginal students can be
afforded a significant chance to attain success.

An unfortunate sidelight exists for programs such as the one described by Henke. Some faculty members, because of their own prejudiced feelings, feel that culturally different students are being given an
advantage they don't deserve by creating such programs. They feel that
extra tutorial and remedial help is a disservice to the student. These
faculty members need to re-examine their reactions to such programs,
and the rationale behind them.

It is vitally important for admissions committees and faculty
members to know and understand the background of individual students. It is difficult to generalize and to anticipate that the previously
stated points will fit all culturally different students; some may not need
such programs, and for others they may be of no significant value. Some
minority group students come from middle-class environments, integrated schools, or school systems that are clearly equal to any. Individual student motives for entrance into the field of nursing, or leaving the field of nursing, must be examined. For example, some culturally different students are hesitant about nursing as a profession because
they feel that nursing is too much a service or subordinate role.

Racism and prejudice are realities which the black and other minority group students must anticipate. Racist practices by fellow students and
by faculty members do exist, although at times they are a little more easily coped with than prejudice or racial practices by the patient. The nursing faculty has an obligation to ensure equal student rights, and, when
deemed necessary, to assist the student in attaining or retaining these
rights. The faculty maintenance of openness, trust, and support will
have significant value for the black student in dealing with her feelings
of insult and the loss of personal and professional worth. Prejudice on
the part of the patient may provide the greater insult, and be the most
difficult for students to resolve. Students will need help through individual and group counseling to understand that an ill patient cannot
be expected to cope with his prejudiced feelings. Patients may send
students out of the room, make disparaging remarks, and so forth. This
is quite discouraging to the culturally different student who sees her
efforts to help rejected. Faculty members must be alert to provide help
to students when this occurs.

## THE OLDER STUDENT

The older student tends to be looked upon with mixed reactions by
faculty members. Some see her as providing the maturity and stability
often lacking in the younger student. Others see her as rigid, and unwilling or unable to learn. Faculty members sometimes find the older
student resentful of accepting supervision from someone younger than

she. As with all other categories of students, the older student must be viewed as an individual rather than classified as a member of a group.

Older nursing students are more likely to be found in schools of nursing requiring less formal education, such as LPN or AD programs. Many are returning to the profession of nursing who started training at one time, stopped for marriage and a family, and are now back to complete a program. Frequently these students have to overcome feelings of inferiority; e.g. they should have gotten their training when they were younger, because now they find it difficult to compete with younger students. Often, family obligations require special consideration so that the student can attend classes. They need help in realizing that the faculty are not interested in having them compete with other students, but rather in helping them to become safe, competent nurses.

The older students present a unique challenge in nursing education in that their life experiences, and personal and social maturation, have pointed out their limitations and achievements. They are surer of who they are and what they want out of life, and consequently tend to have stronger value sets. These value sets may make them less flexible than the job demands. On the other hand, there are many examples of older nursing students who feel too old too learn, who do not have self-confidence, and who consequently may not become effective nurses. Hopefully, these students can be helped through individual and group counseling to become more confident and effective.

Many older students, especially married ones, are still in conflict about their career choice. They have difficulty fitting in with the younger students, or feel that they do. They need periodic reassurance that age does not matter, that their ability and motivation are the important factors. In many areas, such as the ones described earlier in this chapter, the older student has the same problems as the younger student. Nursing educators need to remain alert for those who may need help with particular concerns.

## SUMMARY

In all the situations described in this chapter the emphasis must be placed upon the individual student. It is a mistake for nursing educators to assume common reactions to common situations. The awareness and sensitivity of faculty members will help them identify students in difficulty. Through group discussions, students can be helped to see that they are seldom if ever alone in their feelings or reactions to nursing situations. For almost all the areas discussed in this chapter, group counseling can be an ideal way to meet the needs and concerns of students. This is the subject of our next chapter.

# Chapter 6

# *Group Approaches to Guidance and Counseling*

Up to this point in our discussion of guidance and counseling we have been primarily concentrating on the dyadic or one-to-one relationship. There seems to be little question that provision must be made for individual support for students, particularly in light of the student concerns discussed in the previous two chapters. Nevertheless, we must also recognize that there is currently a great shortage of skilled counselors and psychologists. As a result, there are too few people who have both the skill and the time to meet the demands for individual guidance and counseling. For this reason we are beginning to see the desirability of a rapid expansion in the areas of group guidance and counseling. This new direction holds great promise because of a variety of factors:

1. Group approaches allow for a more rapid and efficient method of information dissemination.

2. They allow students to learn from each other.

3. They are designed to encourage student nurses to learn to use the resources in their peer group. This is an important asset in later functioning as a staff member or leader in team nursing.

4. They allow an individual counselor to come into contact with a much larger group of students than would be feasible on an individual basis.

Group approaches to guidance and counseling are being used at all levels of nursing education today. Although the group techniques used may differ, the general objectives of the group experience seem to remain relatively constant. The purpose of this chapter is to discuss some of the current practices in the use of group approaches in nursing education.

## ORIENTATION PROGRAMS

By far the most prevalent use of orientation programs found in the literature occurs in colleges and universities. Nevertheless the basic principles and organizational structure used in these programs will apply equally well to those schools of nursing not operating in a college setting. It has been found that a well planned orientation program can be a great asset in helping students adjust to their new role as nursing students, in reducing attrition rates, and in serving a diagnostic function to identify those students who may need remedial or tutorial assistance to help them overcome educational deficiencies. There have been tried at least three main approaches to orientation programs. The first of these is the pre-school or precollege summer orientation program; the second is a freshman or new student week prior to the opening of school in the fall; and the third is a continuing weekly orientation program that typically is conducted throughout the first quarter or semester. Let us examine each of these in turn.

The precollege summer orientation program is usually relatively brief and is most commonly found in baccalaureate programs. This concentrated period tends to last two or three days. Two examples come to mind. At Kent State University all freshmen planning to enter school in the fall are required to attend a two-day session during the summer. Their parents are encouraged to attend these sessions with the new students. During the two days the freshmen are given a brief overview of some of the services available to them at the university, such as health services, counseling services, library resources. Parent seminars and tours of campus are held concurrently. After the new students have been provided with the opportunity to talk with college advisors, they are registered for the fall quarter in their appropriate courses. Upperclassmen are actively involved in the program as group discussion leaders. This represents a general orientation to college, with no specific orientation to nursing.

Celano (1969) reports a somewhat different approach in use at the University of Vermont. Here, too, freshmen and transfer students are brought in for a two-day session. During the two days, two hours in the evening and two hours in the morning are devoted to an orientation to nursing. The faculty member who serves as a group leader stresses the need for the development of skills in the areas of communication, leadership, self-directiveness, problem solving, and scholastic interest. In addition, she indicates that regular group meetings will be scheduled during the year. Students have the opportunity to discuss their feelings and raise any unanswered questions. The orientation to nursing and the planned follow-up programs seem to help students to understand the need for related courses and to accept more readily the delay in enrollment in professional classes.

The advantage of the summer preschool or precollege orientation program lies in the fact that all college resources can be mobilized to work with the new students—something that is impossible to do once all the upperclassmen return to school. This time can also be used effectively for guidance testing. There is ample time to have tests scored and remedial plans developed for individual students before they arrive in the fall. Yet there are several disadvantages to this approach. First, it would be desirable to involve upperclassmen in the orientation program as group leaders, tour guides, and the like. They are frequently able to communicate more easily with students on a person-to-person basis. This can also serve as the springboard for a Big Sister program. Nevertheless most upperclassmen are unavailable during the summer, owing to work, family or other obligations. Second, it would be useful to involve as many faculty members as possible in small group interaction with students. Here again, faculty tend to be unavailable during the summer unless they are on 11- or 12-month contracts. Finally, this approach to orientation has its primary usefulness in information dissemination, and helping students get acclimated to their new learning environment. If used as the sole orientation method, it fails to provide an opportunity for students to deal with their personal and professional concerns.

The freshmen week orientation program tries to overcome the disadvantages of the summer program by functioning during the days or week immediately prior to the opening of school in the fall. For example, Boston University requires all incoming freshmen in the School of Education to participate in a three-day session prior to the opening of school. In the past this session was held off campus at a summer camp. During the three days, time was allocated for guidance testing, small group discussions of college life led by upperclassmen with faculty members available as resources, and total group presentations by principal university personnel. Equally important, ample time was allowed for students to interact informally, to get to know each other as members of the new freshman class, and to begin to develop some class cohesiveness.

This approach eliminates the first two problems of the summer orientation program—the unavailability of faculty and upperclassmen—but it fails to solve the problem of dealing with student concerns *as they arise,* particularly during their first quarter or semester in school. As a springboard to a continuing small group discussion session held at regular intervals, it represents a desirable approach. This is especially true because it affords all the advantages of the summer program. In addition, emphasis can be placed on those students who actually intend to enroll in the fall. A percentage of those students who attend summer orientation programs will never reappear for the opening of school. In some cases this is due to multiple college or school applications, and the student's decision to go elsewhere. In other cases personal or family circumstances may change, prohibiting enrollment at this time. In still other cases career objectives may change somewhat, e.g. a baccalaureate student may decide that she prefers an associate degree or diploma program.

The continuing orientation program tends to fall into two parts, the prenursing phase and the concurrent nursing phase. The prenursing phase of continuing orientation applies only to baccalaureate programs that delay admission to the school of nursing until at least the sophomore year. For example, Lun (1966) reports on the program at the University of Hawaii. During the freshman year there are no nursing courses. The nursing faculty have set up small, one-hour, bimonthly meetings with students to discuss employment opportunities, team relationships, advantages and disadvantages of being a nurse, kinds of educational programs in nursing, and expectations of the nursing student. In addition, field trips to hospitals and health services are arranged. Student activities are planned, and a Big Sister program has been developed. A faculty counseling program serves as a referral resource for those students seeking assistance. The faculty have concluded that an orientation program during the first year of a university program is helpful in retaining students' interest in nursing.

By far the most common sort of continuing orientation program is one that functions throughout the students' school or college career and is closely interwoven into the process of nursing education. During the years in the school of nursing, students are continuously involved in orientation to the various clinical areas. The group orientation usually involves a tour of the ward units, an introduction to members of the ward staff, and a discussion of ward policies, routines, procedures, and patient assignments. The students are given information that is felt necessary for them to function comfortably. The same information is given to all the students. Some basic diploma schools affiliate (i.e. send students to other hospitals) for clinical experiences. In such cases the orientation program may be more extensive, since the student needs to become familiar with an entirely different hospital setting.

One of the authors led a student orientation group for affiliating students at a psychiatric hospital. The orientation group was established as a result of a request from the students. They felt the need for some orientation to the hospital prior to their beginning affiliation. Students had heard conflicting stories from other students about the clinical experience. They used the group orientation to talk about what they had seen and what they had expected to see. It proved to be helpful to them in that it alleviated some of their initial anxiety, and they seemed to make a quicker adjustment to the affiliation.

Although the nursing faculty are able to give information to many students in a short period of time, a problem that arises in group orientation is the rapidity with which a large amount of material is given, and the lack of opportunity for the student to participate. The student is not always able to validate the information received or to ask for clarification. When the session is over, students seek each other out for an informal group meeting in the coffee lounge or dormitory in order to compare notes. The informal group may or may not clarify the orientation material disseminated. Some confusion can be eliminated by careful scheduling of the orientation program over longer periods of time. As in the classroom situation, students can absorb only a limited amount of information at any one time. The use of visual aids, hand-outs, role playing, and video tapes makes up for some loss of small group interaction and feedback. Small groups are clearly preferable for orientation because they allow the student a chance to ask questions. Sometimes other students (such as a big sister or brother) can help with the orientation groups. They share their views with the new student, and the new student begins to feel that she has found a friend, someone who has at least lived through orientation. Group orientation should be a learning experience for the students. Kaback (1958) believes that group guidance and counseling are a form of group instruction, and that good teaching techniques are as important in this form of instruction as in regular classroom procedures. The group leader presents information clearly, exhibits an interest in the affairs of the group, and tries to be understanding.

## VOCATIONAL GROUP GUIDANCE IN NURSING EDUCATION

With the increased specialization in nursing, most educators would agree that there is a need for vocational guidance in schools of nursing.

Guidance should be offered early in the student's nursing program so that she can make a wise decision based on adequate information about the myriad kinds of nursing careers. Should she become a staff nurse, a clinician, a private duty nurse? Should she specialize in pediatrics, obstetrics, orthopedics? Should she work in the community, a hospital, a private office, or seek government employment? Should she follow a career in the services? Should she work full or part time? What opportunities are available for nurses in other states and countries? Appropriate answers to these questions cannot be reached until a student has been helped to sort out facts about various careers and her suitability for and interest in them.

Major (1961) points out the need for career guidance in schools of nursing, and career planning with beginning nursing students. She feels that recruitment efforts tend to glamorize nursing, and that faculty members do not adequately guide students toward appropriate career goals. Students need career information that is current and that provides data regarding career opportunities, functions, standards, qualifications, graduate programs, and financial assistance. Schools of nursing have an obligation to assist students in establishing career goals for themselves. Students should fully understand the differences in nursing careers and what is expected of them in specialized fields long before they reach their senior year. Major also pointed out that the attrition from nursing by graduates would decrease if students were helped to plan their futures and find their proper place in the profession.

Graham (1968) reported a study related to graduate work on graduating seniors in 11 programs in nursing in the United States and Canada sponsored by the Seventh Day Adventists. One third of the 266 respondents stated that they planned to enroll in graduate study. Of the total group, 171 made suggestions for guidance to be provided by the schools of nursing and high schools. The findings that support disseminating information regarding graduate study early in the student's career were similar to the results reported earlier by Major. Students requested more in the way of individual vocational counseling. College counseling services do not offer much help in career planning for nursing, and vocational counseling in schools of nursing is often very sketchy, at best.

Prompted by the study done by Major, two senior students at Mt. Sinai Hospital School of Nursing made a study of the career counseling program in their own school. They confirmed, through interviews with 30 students, that when students are enrolled, they have limited knowledge of the functions of a nurse. They also found that at some time during the program, students formulate a goal and an image of a nurse, and that faculty counseling was too little, too late or nonexistent. It would be extremely vital for further research in this area to try to pinpoint the time when students decide on a nursing goal. It is presumed to be midway through the curriculum, and certainly before the senior year.

Students at Mt. Sinai further advocated the employment of a vocational counselor because instructors were either too busy or not adequately prepared. Students also reported that they made decisions about employment based on experiences in the clinical area, readings, discussions with family and classmates, and classes. Since discussions are utilized by students in making vocational choices, and since the number of counselors in nursing available for individuals is limited, it would seem desirable for instructors to provide vocational guidance through groups. Groups would expedite reaching many students and, at the same time, provide an opportunity for students to share their thoughts and feelings about careers with their peers. Students readily share their clinical experiences, and this can provide opportunities for students to hear about a variety of clinical areas without necessarily personally experiencing each one. In this way, group guidance for vocational choices may be even better than the use of individual counseling.

Hewer (1967) conducted a study to evaluate the differential effects of group, individual, and combined group and individual counseling. When realism of vocational choice and satisfaction with employment earnings are used as the criteria for establishing the effectiveness of the three counseling methods, no differences were found. Those students receiving a combination of group and individual counseling expressed greater satisfaction when counseling satisfaction was used as a criterion.

The group approach would seem preferable when a discussion of the merits of each clinical experience related to career development is needed. The individual student may benefit from the support of the group. For example, one student may support another by stating, "I like the way you handle children. They seem to respond warmly toward you." If the student has been thinking about pediatrics as a career, this remark will certainly contribute to her decision. The evidence seems to support the recommendation for ongoing group discussions for student nurses early in their professional career. This method has proved to be successful in schools of nursing. In a group situation the student has several people, including the leader or counselor, who will listen to her, help her understand herself, and provide and validate information that is needed in helping her to make a career decision.

Pallone and Hasinski (1967) found that realism of vocational choice is closely related to the ideal self and occupational role precepts. Therefore knowledge about a career choice in relation to the ideal self-image may have a more powerful influence upon a student's personal satisfaction with a career than congruence between self and ideal self-concepts. Group guidance can certainly be an effective means of providing support, validation, and exchange of ideas with peers in relation to personal satisfaction and vocational choice in nursing.

## EDUCATIONAL GROUP GUIDANCE IN NURSING EDUCATION

Since students tend to be exposed to the group process early in their schooling, it would seem logical that they should purposely and not accidentally learn about group dynamics. Many classes are held in seminar discussions, and educational problems can be solved in a way that permits students to look at how a group functions. A leader is chosen or appointed for each session (sometimes co-leaders are used so that the leaders are more comfortable in the beginning of the learning process), and at the end of the seminar, students look at the group process and leadership. The use of these techniques for teaching students the principles of group process is invaluable in helping them understand the various group roles played by individuals. Hopefully, there is some transfer of learning to other settings, such as clinical patient groups, although this is not viewed as a substitute for formal classwork.

At one university, freshman students meet daily at the end of their clinical experience and discuss their experiences, utilizing group methods. As they begin to function as a group, the instructor initially serves as the leader while each student observes the leadership role. Before the students individually take over the leadership role, they are given assignments outside the class on group process, and have the opportunity to discuss it in class. Both self and peer evaluations of student leadership are utilized. Conferences in many schools of nursing are held at the end of a clinical session, and are handled through group discussion. The foregoing methodology can be used at that time to allow for a further examination of the group process.

Sometimes seminars are structured in a way that allows specific topics to be presented in relation to class material, or they may be entirely dependent on whatever the students want to talk about. In either situation the group process is evaluated. In one psychiatric hospital, students who were affiliating from different schools of nursing were placed in discussion groups for dual purposes: (1) to give them an opportunity to become acquainted and to share feelings about problems; (2) to provide for experimental learning of the dynamics of group process. The students met in groups of 8 to 10, led by a psychiatrist. They were told that their attendance was voluntary, and that they could discuss whatever they liked. They were also told that participation in groups was one way to learn about group process. An instructor acted as recorder and took notes during the sessions. It was explained that the notes were for the purpose of pointing out group process and dynamics. The taking of notes (even though confidential) interfered with spontaneity, but as the group progressed, the recorder was ignored by the students. During group discussions the students talked about problems related to dormitory living, class work and clinical areas, rules and regulations. The psychiatrist did not attempt to deal with unconscious motivations, although students in groups frequently felt that they were being "psyched out" by instructors. The psychiatrist did interrupt the group at various points to help them look at dynamics. At the end of the group sessions, students again were helped to examine the dynamics involved. Written evaluations given by the students were highly in favor of groups, not only for group techniques, but also for their own feelings of satisfaction gained through the group, and through the alleviation of anxiety. Because of their popularity, the group sessions became a regular part of the affiliate program. Later the hospital chaplain led the discussion groups, and the role of recorder was successfully taken over by the students.

Remedial or tutorial groups represent another use of groups in guiding students' educational experience. Students who are experiencing difficulty with certain educational materials may reap benefit by handling such concerns in a group. The group can be helpful to the student in gaining a better understanding of the subject material, improving study habits through exploration of new methods, and giving peer support.

Groups seem to be used successfully in some of the educational programs of nursing schools. The student nurse learns to become a leader of patient groups, such as teaching mothers in obstetrics or diabetics in classes. Since the student nurse can expect to spend many hours in groups as a graduate, it seems logical that the use of groups for guidance and counseling during the nursing program would reinforce the students' skills as they learn to become more comfortable with groups.

## GROUP COUNSELING IN NURSING EDUCATION

The universal use of groups has been closely related to the gregarious nature of man and his herd instinct for survival. Although primitive man did not understand and recognize the dynamics of group process, the group method was basic to his tribal way of life. The stability of "the group" and its survival in modern culture are certainly a testament to a need fulfillment. Man finally got around to the study and identity of group behavior in the nineteenth century (Johnson, 1963). All groups are basically the same, each being structured around a leader and a set of members, with behavior in the group determined by the degree of anxiety produced by the group, which, in turn, is influenced by the amount of closeness in the group (Johnson, 1963).

Group counseling and group therapy are both derived from the more formal group psychotherapy. Group guidance———→group counseling———→group therapy are all on a continuum, differing in degree the same as guidance———→counseling———→psychotherapy differ. All are considered to be processes of learning (Bennett, 1963). Groups can be described as being therapeutic or nontherapeutic. Therapy usually implies that something is wrong with the individual, and treatment is needed to effect a change. Group counseling is thought of more in terms of the group influencing an individual to realize his potentialities and fulfill his ego needs. Groups were first used for therapy by Pratt in the treatment of sick tuberculosis patients. Some nursing educators frown at the mention of group therapy with student nurses, and believe that counselors and educators in schools of nursing are not employed to treat students. If a student is in need of this kind of treatment, then she should be referred. In general, group therapy involves the treatment of emotional illness, group guidance is educationally oriented and concentrates on the imparting of facts, while group counseling emphasizes individual change through learning (Glanz and Hayes, 1967).

Group counseling is effective in helping students deal with their value judgments of patients. Nass and Skipper (1965) found that students bring with them a set of values which affect their relations with patients. Patients who are alcoholics, mentally ill, lack occupational skills, have different skin coloring, and bear illegitimate children are just some of those who are less likely to receive the best care and attention nurses can provide. Students attempting to avoid evaluation and differential treatment of patients require guidance from the nursing faculty and school counselor through group counseling sessions oriented to deal with the problem. With assistance, students can learn to better understand their personal value system and its effect on patients, and provide more effective care.

A similar experience was reported by Yeaworth (1968). She met with 14 students in a maternal nursing course weekly for six weeks. She found that students experience emotional problems when they have to deal with patients whose behavior conflicts with the values held by the students. Group sessions permitted students to verbalize their feelings, learn that others have similar feelings, and share reactions to similar situations. Role playing was ineffective in bringing about new student behavior. Students deny or suppress their feelings out of concern for their patients, and also because of their fear of instructor evaluation. Group counseling thus seems to be an effective way of examining the origin of student attitudes.

Bonner (1959) reported on student nurse reactions to children's deaths at Children's Hospital in Pittsburgh. Students were asked to describe their experiences and reactions to the deaths of patients from ages 5 to 15. She believed that advance preparation for a child's death is needed and can be dealt with effectively in individual or group sessions. Group counseling is an effective way of helping students cope with these painful episodes and learn from them more about themselves and their patients. There are numerous examples of the use of groups in counseling student nurses, and the general agreement is that group counseling does offer an opportunity for positive growth of the self-concept.

Group counseling also provides opportunities for deepened individual insights through the discussion of problems common to the group. Bennett (1963) summarizes four main objectives of group counseling:

1. To provide opportunities for the learning essential for self-direction with respect to educational, vocational, and personal-social aspects of life;
2. To provide an opportunity for the therapeutic effects of group procedures;
3. To achieve some of the objectives of guidance more economically, and some more effectively, than would be possible in a completely individualized approach;
4. To supplement individual counseling and render it more effective through the group study of common aspects of problems and the reduction or elimination of many emotional barriers to the discussion of common problems.

It should be emphasized that group counseling does not take the place of individual counseling if the latter is indicated. In some circumstances the student can be involved in both.

Although schools of nursing have been slow in getting started, nursing educators are now beginning to use and verify the usefulness of group counseling methods. Student nurses who are emerging from the adolescent period of growth and development find that interpersonal feedback from peers, as well as instructors, is vital to their self-concept. As was mentioned earlier, student nurses soon discern that in nursing they are also expected to participate as a member of a variety of groups. In fact, unless she becomes involved in private duty nursing, she will always find herself working in situations in which she is a member of a group.

A survey of recent literature points out the increased use of groups for counseling and guidance in schools of nursing. For example, Golburgh and Glanz (1962) reported on the effectiveness of group counseling in helping college freshmen overcome their difficulty in verbalizing during classroom discussions. They assessed the possibility of change in the quantity of verbalization in classroom discussions through student self-ratings, faculty rating, peer rating, and change in self-attitude in a positive direction as measured by a Self-Attitude Scale. They found that a relatively short period of group counseling has excellent potential for students who have difficulty verbalizing in the classroom. This same approach would apply equally well to other normal concerns of freshmen, e.g. study habits, reading skills, adjustment to college.

Heinemann (1964) reports on the conflicting life and role of a student. She found that freshman students tend to be overwhelmed by their lack of knowledge, and to compare their performance with that of the expert—graduate nurse or their instructor. Their previous life experiences have combined to give them an image of the nurse as viewed by their parents, their teachers, and in some cases, themselves as patients. This image rapidly begins to change when they encounter the reality of patient care and the attitudes of medical and nursing staffs. Through group meetings, students begin to realize that others share the same feelings, and they begin to be able to work through some of their conflicts. This becomes especially important when we recognize that instructors of freshman students serve as role models, and that students frequently tend to treat patients as they have been treated by their instructors.

Culver, Dunham, and Johnson (1963) describe a freshman course at Duke University on Interpersonal Relations. In this particular course, students were encouraged to deal directly with their concerns about patient interaction, and to make every effort to work through their own problems. There proved to be a great deal of group interaction and sharing as the students came to grips with their fears and problems in their gradually increasing involvement in patient care. Although conducted as a course, this experience essentially was a variation of group counseling.

Jordan and Kennedy (1960) reported on a program at the Episcopal Hospital School of Nursing in Philadelphia. A course in Human Relations was developed to assist in the establishment of rapport between the students and the first counselor ever hired by the school. No grades were to be given (an important point for all group experiences) or assignments made. The course content was to be determined primarily by the students. Each student was asked to relate personal problems, although participation in discussion was voluntary and the counselor did not make evaluative statements. The counselor was to be permissive and non-directive, and all discussion was confidential. Principles of group process were discussed as necessary. Sibling rivalry, group deviancy, parental authority, teacher authority, peer group rivalry, boys, rejection, change, marriage as a career, religion, nursing and patients, nursing service and education were all discussed at one time or another. The course was initially extended through the first year; later it was decided to continue the course throughout the three-year program. The authors hope that eventually the course will prove to be unnecessary when the curriculum objective "to make the nurse knowledgeable of feelings" is incorporated throughout the program.

Schultz (1966) reported on the guidance and counseling program at Nebraska Methodist Hospital that has been under the direction of a full-time counselor since 1964. In 1958, when the enrollment doubled to 180 students, it was decided to experiment with the group discussion method with incoming freshmen. Groups of 8 to 12 met with a faculty member at least once a week for 1½ to 2 hours in unstructured sessions. The groups elect their own discussion leaders, the instructors serving as consultants. Discussion topics are presented through a variety of techniques, including role playing, panel presentations, guest speakers, group dynamics, and recommended readings. Two book reports are required relating to personal growth. In addition, each student must write an autobiography and develop a statement of her philosophy of life. Finally, they must complete a personal audit form analyzing their activities, their time and budget allocations, and their satisfying as well as distressing situations. During the second and third years, students meet monthly, with at least every third session unstructured. Through these sessions, students have learned to explore problems of adjusting to independent living. In addition, they begin to learn that each faculty member is also searching for truths, and that it may take a lifetime to know who we are, what we are, what we need, and how to relate to others. In the opinion of the faculty, students seem to mature more rapidly with group counseling, and, as graduates, they seem to have a more perceptive understanding of human relations. Here again, the described experience is a blend of teaching and group counseling techniques; it is much too highly structured to be considered group counseling.

At a Midwest school of nursing, students spend their first year on the college campus, away from the school of nursing. At the end of the year they return to the school of nursing and begin clinical assignments. Students often experience frustration and despair at the change. One director of nursing noted that the change was affecting an entire class, and made arrangements for the students to participate in group counseling. The participation was done on a voluntary basis, under strict rules of confidentiality, and the group was conducted by an educator from outside the school. The students were eager to have a chance to discuss their feelings, many of them related to feelings of inadequacy and inability to live up to the instructor's role models. The group was called a problem-solving group. Among other things, the students presented many problems dealing with dormitory living, for which they used problem-solving techniques. More importantly, students gained the satisfaction of sharing feelings and gaining support from the group. They were able to talk about different clinical areas, and their expectations of the clinical staff, instructors, and co-workers. The group met for a semester, and seemed to feel that it was helpful to talk about concerns and feelings in a group.

Zinberg, Shapiro, and Given (1962) at Beth Israel Hospital in Boston report on the use of Berman's group approach with student nurses and faculty. The purpose of the meetings was to help participants understand something about themselves as people in a professional role, and how they function in a nursing situation. Volunteers were accepted, and sessions were scheduled for 1½ hours over 15 weeks. They found that students' anxiety early in the program was greater than anticipated, but that it gradually decreased with experience.

In a six-year study of satisfaction and stress in nursing programs, Fox et al. (1963) learned that schools of nursing do not encourage enough free and spontaneous communication between students and faculty. They arranged discussion groups over a period of nine weeks in two diploma schools of nursing. They began the discussions by indicating possible topics, although students were told that they could talk about anything they wished. Students reacted favorably when they were given an opportunity to share their feelings and concerns in group discussions.

Kaback (1958) states that although the primary emphasis in group guidance is on content material, the emotional climate created by the group leader often determines whether students experience group participation as group guidance or counseling. In most schools of nursing, counseling is done by an instructor, administrator or faculty advisor. Who, then, is prepared to do group counseling? Group counseling practices are a result of a wide range of applications of counseling theory, and all group practices do not necessarily require rigorous training and experience or developed skill in the use of group dynamics. One can obtain further education and improvement of techniques by participating in groups as either a co-leader or observer. Since many psychiatric nurses are prepared to do group psychotherapy, it would seem likely that some psychiatric nurses could do group counseling well, as could those who have had some training in the use of groups and group discussion. A nurse counselor in a group could also work with a co-leader. Certainly she should have supervision when she does begin group counseling. As was mentioned previously, leadership styles are variable, ranging from free interaction groups to those in which the leader functions with authority. The authors favor a leader who is nondirective, yet able to clarify, guide, and point out relevant material; who is able to help the group look at what is presently happening, and experience growth through problem solving.

The group leader acts as a model for group interaction during the orientation phase of group counseling (Powdermaker and Frank, 1953). In short-term groups a counselor must be prepared to assist students to explore ways of solving problems. For example, one of the writers met with a group of junior students in relation to their feelings about evaluation in the clinical area. Part of their difficulty resulted from their deficiencies in knowing how to study, and part related to the instructor, who they felt demanded perfection in nursing. They had to be helped to solve a communications problem. Students felt that few of them clearly understood the instructor's expectations of them. These students needed help in identifying the real problem, defining related concepts, and finding possible solutions. Many students respond to the complaints of other students by describing similar experiences. Here again, the leader must provide direction by offering comparisons and differences related to the problem. Students may begin with a simple problem that they can identify, share, and for which they can find solutions. Several times in the group, this was done as the leader provided encouragement to follow through with the actions indicated. Reporting the results of the action taken back to the group increased student interest. The group leader facilitates informal learning of participation skills by encouraging democratic patterns of behavior (Gibb et al., 1951). The leader should stress the role of the group members to counteract the feeling that the leader alone is responsible for group outcome. The leader also communicates a feeling of acceptance to each member.

If the leader is expected to relate to individual members as well as the group as a whole, it is important to consider the number of students felt to be ideal for group counseling. A survey of the literature indicates that the group should include 7 to 15 students, although some will suggest from 8 to 10 members. Ideas and perceptions by group members make a significant contribution to the therapeutic process. Too few members limit the amount, variety, and quality of necessary feedback. Too large a group tends to maintain impersonal communication (Kalkman, 1967).

The contract agreed to by the group members and leader establishes policy and control which contributes to the functional structure of the group. It is our feeling through experience and a review of the literature that participation in group counseling ought to be on a strictly voluntary basis, and that sessions should last approximately 1½ hours.

Several other points need to be mentioned in relation to group counseling. It is frequently desirable to maintain written or audio records of counseling sessions. If this is done, these records should be subject to the same guidelines as individual counseling for student nurses. The final point refers to the period through which each group normally moves. The first period is rightfully referred to as the time of orientation. This is the normal period of getting acquainted, testing the limits, establishing the guidelines, and so on. It is a time when each member tries in some way to be the focus of attention. The second period is called the time for working. The group begins to solve problem situations brought in by the group members and leader. The final period is one of termination, and refers to that time when the group has successfully solved problems and achieved a real feeling of group accomplishment.

For those who will be called upon to use group techniques, or to serve as the leader in group counseling sessions, we would refer them to the additional sources identified in the bibliography.

## SENSITIVITY GROUPS IN SCHOOLS OF NURSING

Groups in which the main focus is on the student's feelings, her awareness of them, how she affects others and is affected by them, are known as sensitivity groups. Sometimes these groups are called T-groups or Human Relations training. In the last five years, sensitivity groups have become popular all over the country. A high priority has been given to having students become aware of their feelings, and in all honesty share their feelings with the group. Group members learn to comfortably give feedback as to how they feel about one another.

Some counselors and educators believe in helping students look at their feelings by focusing on a problem or behavior. Others believe in focusing on the students' feelings directly. Having learned to recognize, understand, and deal with one's own feelings will make one better able to live with the self, and make use of the self in relation to others. Again, the group is important because of the necessity to test our feelings and behavior, and to learn how one affects his fellow man.

Some educators believe that sensitization is one way to help students care about others. This is of vital necessity in the helping professions. Some educators and counselors disagree, however, not only as to the value, but also the place, sensitivity groups have in nursing education. There has been minimal research in the area, and much more is needed to lend support to the value of sensitivity training. It is not our intention here to argue on behalf of or against sensitivity training, but rather to examine the pros and cons of the current situation. First, however, we need a closer look at the topic under discussion. Perhaps the best source would be the material issued by the National Training Laboratories for Applied Behavioral Science in 1969. Let us look at some of the questions that have been raised about sensitivity training and the NTL response to them.

1. What is sensitivity training?

Sensitivity training is the currently popular name for a method of experience-based learning originally known as T-group training (the "T" stands for training). There are presently many variations of sensitivity training with names such as encounter groups, personal growth groups, and marathons. In sensitivity training a participant learns human relations, communication, and leadership skills. He learns from his experience in the group by observing and reacting to the behavior (including his own) of group members, under the guidance of a "trainer."

2. What does sensitivity training accomplish?

Most participants gain a picture of the impact they make on other group members. They can compare that impact with their assumptions and intentions, see the range of different perceptions of any given act, discover the common qualities as well as the uniqueness of other individuals, and, if they wish, try out new ways of interacting.

3. What are the qualifications to participate in sensitivity training?

Anyone can participate in sensitivity training if he is free of severe emotional problems and relatively open to learning. It is appropriate for persons of any age.

4. What is the difference between sensitivity training and group therapy?

Sensitivity training is not intended or practiced as a means for correcting significant psychological deficiencies, and persons needing or seeking psychotherapy are discouraged from participating. The incidence of serious stress and mental disturbance during training is difficult to measure. NTL Institute records suggest that fewer than 1 per cent of participants have had significant problems during training under NTL Institute auspices. In almost all cases they have been persons with a history of prior serious disturbances.

5. What are the qualifications of a trainer?

A trainer must have a thorough understanding of group and individual behavior, and skill in using training techniques. He must be in touch with his own feelings, capable of dealing with others in open and nonpunitive fashion, and able to recognize symptoms of severe psychological stress.

With this as a background, let us look more closely at the use of sensitivity training in nursing education. Several schools of nursing have involved their students in T-groups as part of their educational program. Other schools have had their students attend T-groups given by other college departments. Geitgey (1966) did a study of the effects of sensitivity training on the performance of students in associate degree programs of nursing education. She related sensitivity training specifically to the quality of nursing care; interpersonal relations with patients, teachers, and peers; grades in nursing courses; and attrition rates. One hundred and three students in three California junior colleges were subjects for the study. Members of the experimental group experienced sensitivity training while a volunteer control group received instruction in human relations. Statistical findings were significantly favorable at the 0.05 level for the experimental group as measured by patient and instructor evaluation of patient care, and interpersonal relationships with instructors and peers.

Thompson et al. (1965) reported on a process study on sensitivity training and nursing. Results indicated that the sensitivity experience did impel students to look at their behavior and consider areas of needed change. Qualitatively, the process study showed that the students altered their self-concepts as a result of the study. In later interviews the students recommended sensitivity training for other nursing students.

Two students at Hunter College, Daly and Heine (1970), participated in a sensitivity training weekend with other students and faculty. The T-groups consisted of 9 to 12 members. Each of the sessions was different, since they were based on individual experiences. The emphasis in all groups was on honesty and feelings. Verbal and nonverbal means of communication were used in the groups. The students seemed to feel that the purpose of sensitivity training was to learn about oneself and to help others learn about themselves. From the experience the students felt that their communication techniques improved, and that they were able to give better patient care. From this report it seemed that the participants did gain in self-awareness and self-acceptance, while using themselves more fully in their relations with others.

Although a search of the literature shows favorable comments about sensitivity training, it is still not commonly accepted as a necessity in developing the nurse's therapeutic use of self. At one school several nursing students were involved in a marathon weekend T-group. Although feelings ran high and the group was able to express some of them, there was a definite lack of closure as the weekend came to an end. Since some of the feelings were not resolved, they manifested themselves later by disrupting the group cohesiveness of students who were classmates. One of the disadvantages of sensitivity training may be the lack of time needed to work through feelings.

The authors have experienced both positive and negative reactions to sensitivity training. The difference in each case is believed to be based on the qualities of the trainer. More than any other group approach discussed in this chapter, the leader of a sensitivity group must be a skilled, experienced leader in groups. One also questions the soundness of mixing students and faculty together in a sensitivity group. There are many other questions that arise in regard to sensitivity training in nursing education, especially since the area is in great need of substantive research rather than personal bias.

Wyatt (1970) outlined five aspects of any sensitivity program that may be the source of problems. These include the language, the goals, the design, the training staff, and the participants. Wyatt believes that too often there is lack of clarity, misuse and misinterpretation of language. She believes that goals should be clear and specific, and should be written in behavioral terms. The design must be carefully selected, and the training staff must be skillful and knowledgeable. Wyatt further emphasizes voluntary participation, and an appropriate kind of sensitivity training. She concludes with the statement that it is important that proper precautions be taken in setting up a sensitivity program.

Some educators oppose sensitivity groups because they deal too much with the students' feelings. They feel that the student can be harmed psychologically by an inexperienced or unqualified trainer, especially since the group flourishes on reflected self-appraisal. Other educators believe that sensitivity training may be too close to group therapy, and that this treatment of students is inappropriate as part of the educational program.

Unless the school of nursing already has a sound guidance and counseling program for its students in areas of problems, vocations, and so forth, and until more research is done, sensitivity programs in nursing education should be approached in a cautious manner.

# Chapter 7

# *Use of Referral Resources*

Up to this point, Part 1 has described the counseling process, the role of the counselor, the counseling session, and some of the problems presented by students. It has also been emphasized on several occasions that no single counselor can be all things to all students. Inevitably, in the daily work of a faculty member, situations arise with individual students that seem to indicate that referral would be the best course of action. The reader may recall that a counselor is ethically bound to refer a student when she feels that she cannot be of professional assistance, and that the faculty member is not bound to continue the relationship if the student refuses the suggested referral. One of the most difficult questions that must be answered by a faculty member is how, when, and to whom to refer a student who the faculty member feels would benefit by being referred. There is no simple formula for this, no pat answer to fit all situations. Rather, it tends to be highly student-specific and bound by circumstances—the problems presented, the personality variables of both the faculty member and the student, the availability of referral resources, and the timing of the proposed referral. All these are the points to be covered in this chapter. Although we cannot give definitive guidelines to fit all situations, we can explore some alternatives that should prove to be of assistance to a faculty member seeking help in this area.

## WHEN TO REFER

The question of when to refer a student to someone else is a difficult one to answer. It depends on the competency of the counselor, the time she has available, and the evident signs displayed by the student. The first key issue revolves around the point in the counseling relationship at which to introduce the idea of referral. This is the important issue of *timing,* to which we have made reference earlier. If the faculty member introduces the idea of referral too early in the relationship, the student may view her as cold, uninterested, and rejecting. This can be potentially disastrous to the depressed student or the student with a poor self-concept. On the other hand, if the referral comes too late, the faculty member may have fostered a dependent relationship that is difficult to break. With students heading for psychological or other disturbance, waiting too long can greatly increase the severity of the problem and the length and kind of treatment required.

But what is too soon, and what is too late? This question of timing requires professional judgment by the faculty member, for there is no automatic signal which indicates "refer now." Timing refers to that point in the counseling relationship at which the faculty member does something that (a) is neither too soon nor too late, (b) the student is ready for, and (c) the situation calls for. It requires great sensitivity by the faculty member to know when to introduce a new idea or recommendation to a student. The instructor must be very much with the student in her feelings, her understandings, and her awareness of where the student is and where she wants to go.

There are certain guidelines, however, which can be used to help faculty members make a decision about referral. The presence of one or more of these criteria seems to indicate that someone else may be better able to help the student at this time.

1. **At the Request of the Student.**   From time to time a student may introduce the idea of referral herself. In most cases this usually occurs when the student feels that it would be easier for her to talk with someone else outside the school of nursing because of the nature of her problem. The faculty member has to be able to let go in such cases, without feeling hurt or inadequate. The faculty member should check out, however, whether the student really wants referral, or whether she is just testing the faculty member's interest in and commitment to the student and the counseling relationship. This can be done most effectively by exploring with the student the reasons for the referral request, making clear that you are interested in her and in helping her act upon any decision she makes. In order to help her, you need to understand as completely as possible the alternatives available to her, and her feelings about each alternative.

2. **Inability of the Student to Communicate.**   When, after some time, it becomes obvious to you that the student has made no apparent progress and seems to be unable to communicate with you, consideration should be given to having her work with some other person. This is, of course, no indicator of your effectiveness as a counselor, and should not be considered a sign of your own inability, unless it occurs in a significant number of situations. If it does occur frequently, it would seem reasonable that you counsel with someone about your own problem to determine whether you are systematically and unconsciously introducing into the counseling sessions something which interferes with a successful experience.

3. **History of Nervous or Emotional Disorder.**   When it is known or learned that a student has a history of previous emotional disturbance *and* when present symptoms and behavior suggest a gradual deterioration or recurrence, referral is indicated. The fact that the student is coming in to see you may suggest her unwillingness or inability to take the step toward further counseling or therapy. It would not be unreasonable in such cases for you to assist the student by offering to arrange for the referral, or to visit the person to whom she is to be referred with her if necessary or if it would make her more comfortable.

4. **When the Faculty Member Feels a Personal Bias or Barrier Which Is Interfering with the Professional Relationship She Should Be Providing for a Student.** At times the faculty member may find that she is uncomfortable working with a particular student because of her own biases, the nature of the student's problem, or some idiosyncracy or physical characteristic of the student which creates problems for the faculty member. At the other end of the continuum, the faculty member may begin to realize that she has become too emotionally involved with the student, to the extent that she can no longer maintain the helping relationship on a professional level. In either case, referral is indicated.

5. **When the Nature of the Student's Concern May Require More Time than the Faculty Member Is Able to Devote Because of Her Other Responsibilities.** This is perhaps the most common reason for referral. The faculty member may feel that the student will need long-term treatment. Some students make excessive demands on a faculty member's time by requesting appointments, which may be useful or necessary for her, two or three times a week. The greater the number of students for whom the faculty member has responsibility, the less able is she to provide such intensive and extensive assistance. It must also be recognized that most faculty members lack the professional training and experience to provide long-term treatment. In such cases the student is better referred to someone else.

## REFERRAL TO WHOM?

When a faculty member has reached the point at which she feels that referral is indicated, she must immediately begin to consider both what is available in the way of referral resources, and which one of these would be best for the student with whom she is working. The first part of this consideration should be answered by already available information gathered by a counselor or student-faculty guidance committee. There are several approaches to the question of to whom to refer. The first is to move through a gradually more sophisticated chain of resources in which the student is simply referred to the next level. The second is to select the most appropriate referral resource from a group of those available. Both approaches are workable. The first would probably be better for relatively unsophisticated faculty members who hesitate to diagnose, and who are unsure of where a student should be sent. The second would be more likely to be used by an experienced counselor.

The list of available resources will vary somewhat, depending on the school of nursing, the college, the community, and the surrounding area. Perhaps the best way to explain the normal flow of a student referral would be to use an open-ended systems analysis approach.

In block 1.0 of Illustration on p. 94 the student is in need of referral as seen by herself or others in the school on the basis of her academic performance, clinical practice or personal-social interaction. Either alone or with assistance, the student gathers and analyzes the available information and decides on the best referral resource. On the basis of the data analysis, the student is then referred to one of the initial services in the second block.

In block 2.0 the student is seen by one or more of the initial services, which include nursing educators, chaplain, physician, and college counseling center. The referral agent assesses the needs of the student and proceeds to work with her in the area of concern. At the appropriate time the student and the referral agent decide together whether the needs of the student have been met. If so, the services provided are terminated. If not, the student is referred to one of the specialized services in the next block.

In block 3.0 the student is again seen by one or more specialized services such as psychiatrist or psychologist, physician or other specialist. Again, the referral agent at this level assesses the needs of the student and proceeds to work with her in the area of concern. At the appropriate time the student and the specialist decide together whether the needs of the student have been met. If so, the services provided are terminated. If not, the student is referred to one of the specialized settings in the next block.

In block 4.0 the student enters a specialized center for a particular need such as drug abuse, abortion, community mental health. The referral agent at this level assesses the need and works with the student. At the appropriate time the student and the center resource person evaluate the outcomes. If these are deemed to be adequate, the services are terminated. If they are deemed to be inadequate, the student is recycled into block 2.0 to begin seeking once again other sources of help.

If, at any time after services have been terminated, the student is again in need of assistance for any reason, she once again enters the system and continues until she gets the appropriate help for the concern she is expressing. This diagram of an open system is not meant to include all possible resources that may be available to students and faculty in a school of nursing. Others found to be useful may be incorporated at the appropriate level. In addition, the system will need to be regularly reexamined to ensure that it is still serving the function for which it was designed—a systematic method of providing the appropriate services to students in need of help.

To reiterate, one of the first jobs of a new counselor or of a newly created or revitalized student-faculty guidance committee is to conduct a careful and complete analysis of all possible resources available to students. This analysis should include the following types of information:
1. Name, address, and telephone number of resource
2. Kinds of problems handled
3. Availability of appointment
4. Fee, if any
5. Kinds of information requested with referral
6. Kinds of information that will come back to source of referral, if any.
Such an analysis should be regularly rechecked for accuracy. It should also be carefully summarized and placed in the hands of students as part of an orientation to counseling.

A SYSTEMS APPROACH TO STUDENT REFERRAL

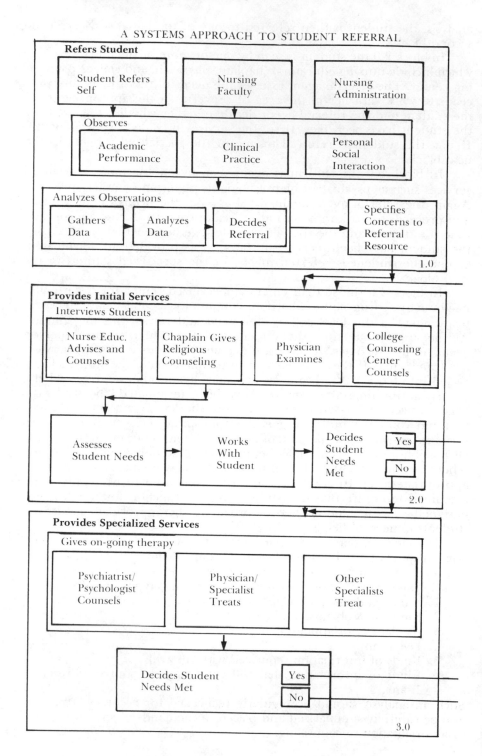

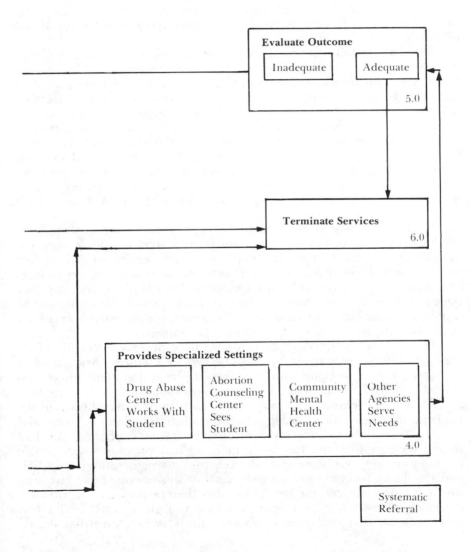

## HOW TO REFER

The third, and perhaps the most important, question deals with the problem of how to refer. Arranging for a student to accept the idea of seeing someone else is at best a tricky situation. Frequently the suggestion of referral produces unforeseen reactions on the part of a student. Each of these reactions challenges the ingenuity and sensitivity of the faculty member, and must be dealt with very specifically if the referral is to be accepted by the student. Possible reactions include the following:

1. "You must think that I'm really sick if you want me to see someone else." This puts many faculty members on the defensive, since they don't wish to frighten off the student by a "Yes" response. On the other hand, a negative response may cause the student to terminate without recognizing the seriousness of desirability of referral. In general, explaining to the student as clearly as possible why you recommend referral will usually forestall this response.

2. "Why must I start over with someone else just when I've gotten to know you?" A variation to this would be, "After telling you things that I've never been able to tell anyone else, I don't think I can or want to start over again with someone new." In both cases the faculty member tends to be greatly flattered by the student's response, and it is not unusual for a faculty member to agree to continue working with a student even though she professionally believes that referral would have been best. These reactions might best be handled by reinforcing and supporting the student's ability to talk with someone else, the faculty member's caring for the student as a reason for referral, and perhaps offering to go with the student to meet the new counselor or therapist if the student is too fearful.

3. "I might have known you would reject me just like everyone else has." This is not an unusual response from a student with a very low self-concept or one who is quite depressed. Here again, strong support by the faculty member is indicated. This response usually triggers feelings of guilt and inadequacy in faculty members. They begin to feel that they have failed the student. None of these feelings is valid, but they must be understood and not allowed to turn the instructor's empathy into sympathy so that professional judgment becomes impaired.

Perhaps the outstanding example we have observed recently of an excellent referral was made by a young faculty member in a school of nursing. She was working with a severely depressed student nurse who she felt required a level of assistance far more sophisticated than the help she felt able to provide. She introduced the idea of referral once to the student, and the student asked why she couldn't continue to work with the faculty member, since she had already started with her, she had shared feelings with the instructor that she had previously felt unable to communicate to anyone else, she felt the instructor understood her, and she didn't feel able to start over again with someone new. Listening carefully to the student, the faculty member then responded, "If you were extremely interested in a patient of yours, and giving care, and knew, in your heart, that you couldn't give her the very best care that she required, would you not feel it better to go get someone who could give the care the patient required?" In her response, given in a calm yet warm and empathic voice, the counselor communicated deep concern, sensitivity, understanding, and, above all, genuine caring, all in a relatively brief, simple response. This is not meant to suggest that the response is ideal for all situations; no single response is universally ideal. Nevertheless the ingredients of this response ideally should be part of any referral process.

## SOME GENERAL OBSERVATIONS

Several general considerations relating to the process of referral are worth discussing briefly.

1. **Making the Referral Contact.**   As a general rule, in guidance and counseling, it is desirable to encourage student initiative and responsibility at every opportunity. For example, it is better to indicate sources of information for a student, and encourage her to take the initiative in seeking them out. The same principle holds true in the referral process, i.e. indicating sources of help available to the student, and encouraging her to take the initiative in utilizing one or more of them. But in referral situations in which the student is experiencing great difficulty getting up enough courage to utilize the referral source, the faculty member may wish to (a) make the appointment for the student, if she is sure the student wants this, and (b) go with the student to introduce her to the new counselor or other resource in order to facilitate transfer. Either or both of these approaches may be used if they will facilitate satisfactory referral.

2. **Transmission of Information.**   Frequently it is difficult for a faculty member to know how much information about a referred student to give the new counselor or other specialist. As a general rule, this should be discussed first with the student. Some students feel more comfortable starting fresh with a new counselor. Others would prefer the faculty members to talk to the new counselor, especially if they know what the faculty member is going to say. No information should be given to the new counselor or agency without the student's knowledge and permission. This is true of both written and verbal communications; the only exception would be the situation in which consultation with the student is impossible because of severe emotional disturbance. The faculty member should also be aware that some referral sources will neither want nor accept any information about a student; the new resource prefers to start from scratch, with as few biases as possible, forming her own opinions. If such is the case, and if the student is expecting her history and problem to be transmitted, this should be communicated to the student.

3. **If the Referral Is Refused.**   We have already stressed the facts that (a) the faculty member is ethically under no obligation to continue the counseling relationship if the referral is refused, and that (b) the faculty member must decide whether her help on a continuing basis is better or worse than the student's receiving no further assistance because she refuses to be referred. Two additional points should be stressed. If the

faculty member has attempted to refer, been refused by the student and therefore has agreed to continue working with the student so that the student will at least get some help, the instructor then has two obligations:

    a. To consult regularly with another professional for support in her approach to counseling the student. This is particularly important if the original reason for referral was based on the felt inadequacy of the faculty member.

    b. To remember constantly that she now has a new primary objective in counseling, i.e. to help the student reach the point at which she will accept the idea of referral. The original reasons for referral will in all likelihood remain, so that the instructor should continue to try to bring the student to the point of referral.

    4. **Permission for Referral or Consultation.** As a general rule, parental permission is unnecessary for a referral. This is particularly true with the age group we are working with among student nurses. If, however, the counselor is obligated to obtain parental permission before any referral takes place, or a specific kind of referral occurs, because of school or other policy, under no circumstances should any parental contact be made without the prior knowledge and permission of the student. Such a violation of confidence by a faculty member will in all probability not only destroy her relationship with the individual student concerned, but also greatly impair her future effectiveness with other students. A reputation for trustworthiness and confidentiality takes time for a faculty member to build. Such a reputation can be impaired or destroyed quickly by any violation of this trust or confidence. This same principle applies to administrative permission for a referral. If the faculty member is required to obtain approval from or to communicate with an administrator within the school, this limitation should be carefully explained to the student as early as possible, as should any other limitation to the confidentiality of the counseling relationship.

    5. **After the Referral Has Been Made.** One of the most frustrating things for an instructor or counselor to accept is the lack of feedback from a referral source about a student once a referral has been made. Frequently the faculty member has developed a deep interest in the student, and wishes to know not only how the new relationship is going, but also if she can be of additional help. It must be remembered that the new counselor or agency is also bound by the rules of confidentiality, and cannot feed such information back to the referring source. Occasionally the student herself will drop in and let the faculty member or counselor know how things are going. This generally is the only source of information that can and will be forthcoming. The faculty member and counselor should not interpret this as a lack of trust in her, but rather as a reflection of the ethical restriction on the new counselor or agency.

    6. **Dual Counseling.** Occasionally a situation may arise in which a referral is made successfully, but the student wishes to continue working also with the original instructor or counselor. Sometimes an instructor counsels, refers the student, and then continues to see the student in the classroom or clinical area as part of her normal instructional re-

sponsibilities. This is not dual counseling; we are referring here to the instructor who counsels, refers, and continues to counsel at the same time the student is being seen by someone else. This should be avoided if at all possible because of the likelihood of working at cross purposes with the new counselor or agency. If for some reason such an arrangement seems likely to occur, two conditions must be met:

a. The purpose of counseling should be sharply different from that of the new counselor or agency; e.g. the new resource is working with personal problems of adjustment, while the original counselor or instructor continues to work with career information or educational guidance.

b. Continual consultation should go on between both counselors to ensure compatibility, and mutual agreement must be arrived at between both counselors before entering into such an arrangement. Some counselors or agencies will refuse to work with a student who is seeing someone else at the same time unless they are convinced that the other counselor will in no way interfere with the therapeutic relationship.

7. **The Safety Valve.** Another common trap for a faculty member occurs when a student is shaky about accepting a referral. In an effort to convince the student, the instructor sometimes suggests that the student try the new counselor, and if she isn't happy with the new relationship, the student is welcome to return once more to the original counselor. Such an escape clause should not be provided for several reasons:

a. It places the new counselor in the difficult position of not having a student committed to developing a new counseling relationship.

b. The original reason for referral still exists; the original counselor either is in no better position to provide the kind of help needed by the student, or the original reason for referral was invalid.

c. Such a suggestion encourages dependency by the student on the faculty member, and also indicates a faculty member who is afraid or unable to let go of the student because of emotional involvement, feelings of guilt about the referral, or for other reasons.

8. **The Shopping Client.** Every once in a while we come into contact with the student who shops around for psychological assistance, freely and quickly moving from resource to resource, in general talking with anyone who will listen to her. This pattern may occur in a very dependent student, in a student who will never deal with her real concerns, for she jumps to a new counselor whenever the old one begins to get too close, or in a student who is undergoing counseling for experience, but with no real commitment to any personal investment. A faculty member or counselor should not agree to work with a student, or accept a referral of a student, unless she is satisfied that the student not only wishes counseling assistance, but also is willing to invest the personal energy necessary to help the counseling relationship develop. Essentially, we must remember that we have neither the time nor the personnel to provide a psychological supermarket for students.

Referral is never an easy process; not uncommonly it can prove to be a very difficult experience for both the faculty member and the student. It may produce feelings of rejection, threat, and anxiety on the part of the student. Each may have great difficulty letting go of the other. Yet the faculty member who truly has the best interest of the student at heart, and who is able to recognize objectively what is best for the student regardless of personal feelings, will never hesitate to refer the student to someone else when she no longer feels able to help.

# BIBLIOGRAPHY

*Part 1*

Aldag, Jean C.: Occupational and Non-Occupational Interest Characteristics of Men Nurses. *Nursing Research,* Vol. 19, No. 6, November-December, 1970.

Aldag, Jean C., and Christensen, Cheryl: Personality Characteristics of Male Nurses. *Nursing Research,* Vol. 16, No. 4, Fall, 1967.

Baker, Carl G.: Quoted by Harry Nelson. *Honolulu Advertiser,* 23 April 1971, p. A-15.

Barckley, Virginia: Enough Time for Good Nursing. *Nursing Outlook,* Vol. 12, No. 4, April, 1964, p. 44.

Becker, Howard S.: On Becoming a Marijuana User. *The Outsiders.* Free Press of Glencoe, 1963.

Bell, Gordon R.: *Escape from Addiction.* New York, McGraw-Hill Book Company, Inc., 1970.

Benjamin, Alfred: *The Helping Interview.* Boston, Houghton Mifflin Company, 1961.

Bennett, Margaret E.: *Guidance and Counseling Groups.* 2nd ed. New York, McGraw-Hill Book Company, Inc. (Series in Guidance, Counseling and Student Personnel in Education), 1963.

Blaine, Graham B., and McArthur, Charles C.: *Emotional Problems of the Student.* 2nd ed. New York, Appleton-Century-Crofts, Inc., 1971.

Bonner, Hubert: *Group Dynamics.* New York, Ronald Press Co., 1959.

Bowers, Margaretta, Jackson, Edgar N., Knight, James A., and LeShan, Lawrence. *Counseling the Dying.* New York, Thomas Nelson and Sons, 1964.

Brainerd, Franklin: Rather than Scream. *Today's Health,* June, 1971.

Brammer, Lawrence M., and Shostrom, Everett: *Therapeutic Psychology.* Englewood Cliffs, N.J., Prentice Hall, 1960.

Brauer, Paul H.: Should the Patient Be Told the Truth? *Nursing Outlook,* Vol. 8, December, 1960, p. 672.

Brown, Norman K., Thompson, Donovan J., Bulger, Roger J., and Laws, E. Harold: How Do Nurses Really Feel About Euthanasia and Abortion? *American Journal of Nursing.* Vol. 71, No. 7, July, 1971, pp. 1413–1416.

Burton, Genevieve: The Instructor-Counselor. *Journal of Nursing Education,* Vol. 1, No. 4, December, 1962, pp. 5–10.

Celano, Paula Johnson: A Prefreshman Orientation Program. *Nursing Outlook,* Vol. 17, No. 6, June, 1969, p. 84.

Cleland, Virginia: Sex Discrimination: Nursing's Most Pervasive Problem. *American Journal of Nursing,* Vol. 71, No. 8, August, 1971, pp. 1542–1547.

Coleman, Kevin: Student Attitudes Re: Drugs. Unpublished Survey, Kent State University, Ohio, 1971.

Commonly Asked Questions About Sensitivity Training and NTL Institute. *NTL Institute News and Reports,* June, 1969.

Culver, Charles, Dunham, Frances, and Johnson, Betty: A First Course in Interpersonal Relations. *Nursing Forum,* Vol. 2, No. 1, January, 1963, pp. 79–85.

Daly, Nancy Ann, and Heine, Hildy Corinne: Honesty Is the Secret in Sensitivity Training. *Nursing Outlook,* Vol. 18, No. 6, June, 1970, pp. 36–39.

Deutch, Martin, Katz, Irwin, and Jensen, Arthur: *Social Class, Race, and Psychological Development.* New York, Holt, Rinehart and Winston, 1968.

Drug Abuse: Escape to Nowhere. Philadelphia, Smith, Kline and French Laboratories, 1967.

Elmore, James L., and Verwoerdt, Adrian: Psychological Reactions to Impending Death. *Hospital Topics,* Vol. 45, November, 1967, p. 315.

Ethical Standards, APGA. Washington, D.C., American Personnel and Guidance Association, 1961.

Feder, Daniel D.: Selection and Training of Faculty Counselors; in E. G. Williamson (Ed.): *Trends in Student Personnel Work.* Minneapolis, University of Minnesota Press, 1949.

Feifel, Herman: *The Meaning of Death.* New York, McGraw-Hill Book Company, Inc., 1959.

Fonseca, Jeanne D.: Induced Abortion. *American Journal of Nursing,* Vol. 68, No. 5, May, 1968, pp. 1022–1027.

Fosberg, Gordon C.: Men Nurses Are There in Air Evacuation. *American Journal of Nursing,* Vol. 69, No. 2, February, 1969, pp. 312–315.

Fox, David J., Diamond, Lorraine K., Knapf, Lucille, Walsh, Ruth, and Hodgin, Jean: Can "Just Talking" Be Planned? *American Journal of Nursing,* Vol. 63, No. 8, August, 1963, pp. 107–110.

Geitgey, Doris Arlene: A Study of Some Effects of Sensitivity Training on the Performance of Students in Associate Degree Programs of Nursing Education. Unpublished Doctoral Dissertation, University of California at Los Angeles, 1966.

Gibb, J. R., Platt, Grace R., and Miller, L. F.: *Dynamics of Participation in Groups.* St. Louis, John F. Swift Co., 1951.

Giffen, Kim: Interpersonal Trust in the Helping Profession. *American Journal of Nursing,* Vol. 69, No. 7, July, 1969, pp. 1491–1492.

Glanz, Edward C., and Hayes, Robert W.: *Groups in Guidance.* 2nd ed. New York, Allyn and Bacon, 1967.

Golburgh, Stephen J., and Glanz, Edward C.: Group Counseling with Students Unable to Speak in Class. *Journal of College Student Personnel,* Vol. 4, No. 2, December, 1962, pp. 102–103.

Graham, Lois E.: Are We Motivating Students to Go on for Graduate Education? *Nursing Outlook,* Vol. 16, No. 8, August, 1968, pp. 48–50.

Heinemann, M. Edith: The Conflicting Life of a Student. *Nursing Outlook,* Vol. 12, No. 3, March, 1964, pp. 35–38.

Henke, St. Grace: Project Tap—A Tutorial Program. *American Journal of Nursing,* Vol. 71, No. 5, May, 1971, pp. 978–981.

Hewer, Vivian H.: Evaluation of Group and Individual Counseling: A Follow-up. *Journal of College Student Personnel,* Vol. 8, No. 4, July, 1967, pp. 265–270.

Jensen, Arthur Robert: *Individual Differences in Learning: Interference Factor.* Berkeley, University of California Press, 1964.

Johnson, James A.: *Group Therapy: A Practical 1963 Approach.* New York, McGraw-Hill Book Company, Inc., 1963.

Jordan, Clifford H., and Kennedy, Jane: Counseling That Enriches. *American Journal of Nursing,* Vol. 60, No. 2, February, 1960, pp. 231–233.

Kaback, Goldie: *Guidance and Counseling Perspectives for Hospital Schools of Nursing.* New York, N.L.N., 1958.

Kalkman, Marian E.: *Psychiatric Nursing.* New York, McGraw-Hill Book Company, Inc., 1967.

Kubler-Ross, Elizabeth: *On Death and Dying.* London, Macmillan Company, Collier-Macmillan, 1969.

Kubler-Ross, Elizabeth: Seminar for the Terminal Patient. *Roche Medical Image and Documentary,* Vol. 11, No. 6, December, 1969, p. 20.

Lingeman, Richard R.: *Drugs from A to Z: A Dictionary.* New York, McGraw-Hill Book Company, Inc., 1969.

Lun, Jean J.: A Freshman Orientation Program. *Nursing Outlook,* Vol. 14, No. 4, April, 1966, pp. 36–37.

McGrath, Joseph E., and Scarpitti, Frank R.: *Youth and Drugs; Perspectives on a Social Problem.* Chicago, Scott, Foresman and Company, 1970.

Major, Dorothy: Career Guidance Needed in Nursing Schools. *Nursing Outlook,* Vol. 9, No. 9, September, 1961, pp. 536–537.

Major, Dorothy: Career Planning Begins with the Beginning Student. *Nursing Outlook,* Vol. 9, No. 9, September, 1961, pp. 534–536.

Maslow, Abraham: *Motivation and Personality.* New York, Harper and Row, 1954.

Massachusetts Nurses State Right of Refusing Tasks on Grounds of Conscience. *American Journal of Nursing,* Vol. 71, No. 9, September, 1971, p. 1668.

Nass, Gilbert D., and Skipper, James K.: The Value Judgment Dilemma in Patient Care. *Nursing Outlook,* Vol. 13, No. 6, June, 1965, pp. 33–35

Nehren, Jeanette, and Killen, Barbara: Preventive Counseling for Nursing Students. *Nursing Outlook,* Vol. 15, No. 1, January, 1967, pp. 37–39.

N.L.N. Measurement and Evaluation Service: Let's Examine Attrition Rates in Schools of Nursing. *Nursing Outlook,* Vol. 18, No. 9, September, 1970, p. 58.

Orlando, Ida Jean: *The Dynamic Nurse-Patient Relationship.* New York, Putnam, 1961.

Pallone, Nathaniel, and Hasinski, Marian: Reality-Testing a Vocational Choice: Congruence Between Self, Ideal and Occupational Percepts Among Student Nurses. *Personnel and Guidance Journal,* Vol. 45, No. 7, March, 1967, pp. 666–670.

Powdermaker, F., and Frank, J.: *Group Psychotherapy.* Cambridge, Harvard University Press, 1953.

Quint, Jeanne C.: *The Nurse and the Dying Patient.* New York, Macmillan Company, 1967.

*Rehabilitation of the Narcotic Addict.* Report of the Institute on New Developments in the Rehabilitation of the Narcotic Addict. Fort Worth, Texas, 1966.

Rhoads, Paul S.: *Management of the Patient with Terminal Illness,* The Journal of the American Medical Association, Vol. 192, No. 8, May 24, 1965, p. 662.

Riesman, David: *The Lonely Crowd.* New Haven, Yale University Press, 1967.

Rogers, Carl: *On Becoming a Person.* Boston, Houghton Mifflin Company, 1961.

Schultz, Charlotte Rees: New Dimensions in a Guidance Program. *Nursing Outlook,* Vol. 14, No. 5, May, 1966, pp. 56–57.

Somerville, Rose M.: Death Education as Part of Family Life Education; Using Imaginative Literature for Insights into Family Crises. *The Family Coordinator,* Vol. 20, No. 3, July, 1971, p. 209.

Stephens, Gwen: Mind-Body Continuum in Human Sexuality. *American Journal of Nursing,* Vol. 70, No. 7, July, 1970, pp. 1468–1471.

Thompson, Vaida D., Lakin, Martin, and Johnson, Betty Sue: Sensitivity Training and Nursing Education: A Process Study. *Nursing Research,* Vol. 14, No. 2, Spring, 1965, pp. 132–137.

Verwoerdt, Adrian, and Wilson, Ruby: Communication with Fatally Ill Patients—Tacit or Explicit. *American Journal of Nursing,* Vol. 67, No. 11, November, 1967, pp. 2307–2309.

Whitaker, Dorothy, and Lieberman, Martin A.: *Psychotherapy Through the Group Process.* Englewood Cliffs, N.J., Prentice Hall, 1964.

Wyatt, Wendy C.: Responsible Use of Sensitivity Training. *Nursing Outlook,* Vol. 18, No. 6, June, 1970, pp. 39–40.

Yeaworth, Rosalie: Mental Health: A Two-Way Street. *Nursing Outlook,* Vol. 16, No. 11, November, 1968, pp. 45–48.

Zinberg, Norman, Shapiro, David, and Gruen, Walter: A Group Approach to Nursing Education. *Nursing Outlook,* Vol. 10, No. 11, November, 1962, pp. 744–746.

# Part 2

# *Evaluation*

# Chapter 8

# Introduction to Measurement

Although the present chapter is concerned primarily with measurement, an initial discussion of evaluation will be presented to build a rationale for the critical part measurement plays in the maintenance of sound educational practices in a school of nursing. The body of the chapter will contain basic concerns of measurement.

Evaluation as an integral part of nursing education has received considerable attention during recent years. Although emphasis has been placed on innovative approaches, such as the application of behavioral objectives to the educational process, the nursing educator's evaluation of student progress is still heavily based upon subjective judgment. This judgment is often aided by questionable interpretation of data obtained from questionably constructed measuring devices. Perhaps student evaluation will always have a degree of subjectivity on the part of the educator-evaluator; however, it is the intent of the present chapter to provide a rationale for the development of a sound objective basis for student evaluation.

The intent of the chapter cannot be carried out without concern for the effectiveness of the nursing school, its guiding philosophy, and operational hypotheses. Although chapter 15 covers the specific recommendations of the authors, it may be useful to reiterate evaluation concerns. It may also be necessary to examine assumptions on which an evaluation might be based. Does the nursing program see education as a process which seeks to change the behavior patterns of students? To what extent are the desired changes part of the educational objectives of the nursing educational program? In what way are the behavior patterns organized, and how are they to be appraised for effectiveness? Are the methods for student evaluation limited to paper-and-pencil achievement tests or is any other device or situation used to provide valid data on progress toward achieving educational objectives? To what extent are nursing educators, clinical staff, and the student equal participants in the process of evaluation?

It appears essential that a formulation of an evaluation program, including purpose and basic assumptions, be clearly agreed upon. Within this framework the units of the learning situation as well as the behavioral and educational objectives should be formulated, classified, and clearly stated.

## EDUCATIONAL AND BEHAVIORAL OBJECTIVES

Statements of objectives are most clearly defined in terms of learner behavior. If one is to obtain data pertinent to the behavioral objectives, it is also necessary to specify the situation in which the behavior is to be demonstrated: classroom, bedside, laboratory or social settings. Obtaining valid data is perhaps the most important step in the evaluation procedure. Evaluators should bear in mind that the most thorough evaluation procedures utilize various evaluation tools. In addition to formalized tests, interviews, observations, questionnaires, and ratings may also provide valid data for determining the degree to which desirable changes in behavior patterns of the learner are occurring. Depending upon the nature of the measurement tasks, nursing educators may find ready-made measurement instruments or, more likely, may find no measurement instrument available to measure certain objectives. It is the contention of the authors that the more clearly stated are the objectives, goals, and testable assumptions for a nursing program, the easier is the task of measuring achievement for each student. Let us examine some of the characteristics of behavioral objectives.

An objective is an intent communicated by a statement describing a proposed change in a student, a statement of what the student is to be like when she has successfully completed a learning experience. It is a description of a pattern of behavior (performance we want the student to be able to demonstrate).

Another characteristic requirement is clearly defined goals or terminal behaviors, followed by the evaluation of the degree to which the student is able to perform in the manner desired (meeting a criterion). An additional advantage of clearly defined objectives is that the student is provided the means to evaluate her own progress at any place along the route of instruction and is able to organize her efforts into relevant activities.

Objectives are meaningful to the extent that they convey to the student a picture identical to that which the writer of the objective has in her mind. The effectively stated objective is one that succeeds in communicating your intent and excludes the greatest number of possible unintended alternatives to the goal. The statement, then, that communicates is the one that describes the terminal behavior (what the student will be doing to demonstrate fullfillment of the objective) well enough to minimize misinterpretation.

Mager (1961) presents a three-stage scheme as a guide to writing behavioral objectives:

1. Identify the terminal behavior by name; you can specify the kind of behavior that will be accepted as evidence that the learner has achieved the objective.
2. Try to define the desired behavior further by describing the important conditions under which the behavior will be expected to occur.
3. Specify the criteria of acceptable performance by describing how well the learner must perform to be considered acceptable. Terminal criteria may be time limits, minimum number, percentage, minimum acceptable skill level, minimal acceptable accuracy or deviations.

The foregoing does not do justice to the highly developed area of educational and behavioral objectives. The reader is encouraged to read

Mager's text as well as those written by Armstrong et al. (1970) and Silvern (1968).

Eisner, cited by Treece (1970), raises four limitations to using educational objectives. First, owing to the dynamic interaction of numerous instructional styles and outcomes, it is difficult to specify behavior and content items in advance. Second, the uniqueness of the subject matter may place unrealized constraints on behavioral objectives. Third, a possible faulty assumption that objectives can be used as standards by which to measure achievement fails to distinguish adequately between application of the standard and the making of judgment. Fourth, identifying the objectives prior to proceeding to identify activities may be logically defensible, but not necessarily psychologically efficient. Also, empirical evidence is lacking to demonstrate significant changes in teaching, learning or curriculum building.

The fourth limitation is open to question, in that if behavioral objectives are not to mislead the student, they must be stated in terms of activities to be performed. Objectives are stated in specific behaviors the student is to demonstrate if she is to satisfy an objective. If we focus on specific outcomes as indicated by student behavior, then the appropriateness and adequacy of our teaching can be more easily determined. We will then have a sounder basis from which to evaluate student progress and the effectiveness of the experiences provided students.

The presentation up to now has used educational objective as synonymous with "behavioral objective," although some readers as well as writers would not agree. "Educational objectives" may be perceived to be a more inclusive term and include a series of behavioral objectives which, when summed or combined, would demonstrate an educational objective. A number of recent attempts have been made to clarify and further develop the concept of educational objectives. One of the most comprehensive of these efforts is that which resulted in the publication of the Taxonomy of Educational Objectives (Bloom, 1956; Krathwohl, 1964). The taxonomy attempts to classify all the various kinds of educational objectives:

1. *Cognitive objective,* which are those dealing with remembering, recognizing knowledge, the development of intellectual abilities and skills, and so forth.
2. *Affective objectives,* which are those dealing with interests, attitudes, opinions, appreciations, values, emotional sets, and so forth.
3. *Psychomotor objectives,* which are those involving the development of muscular skills, coordination, and so forth.

The Taxonomy of Educational Objectives may be of help to educators in maintaining perspective on the relative emphasis they are giving to certain kinds of learning. In summary, the following principles concerning educational objectives may be useful as guides to the nursing educator:

1. Define for each course or class the specific objectives used to provide direction for daily instruction.

2. These specific objectives should be consistent with the more general objectives of the nursing faculty.

3. Educational objectives are best stated in terms of observable student behavior so that progress toward the objectives can be measured.

4. The specified objectives should assess a variety of different kinds of learning.

5. Objectives should be stated as actions simply, specifically, and clearly.

6. Each item or behavior of a test or assessment instrument should be directly related to one of the educational objectives of the course.

## MEASUREMENT

Measurement has always been susceptible to two kinds of error: errors due to limitations in the measuring instruments, and errors in the administration of the instruments.

The terms "measurement" and "evaluation" are often incorrectly used as synonyms in spite of the fact that they are distinctly different processes. Measurement is viewed as routine and objective, while evaluation is viewed as intellectual and subjective. Measurements are seldom taken without premeasurement specifications of purpose or evaluation of the results. Measurement is the application of an instrument or instruments to collect data for some specific purpose. Evaluation is the process of subjective appraisal with specific purposes or aims in mind. This appraisal begins with the data or information which has been collected through the measurement process. Measurement does not guarantee relevant evaluation, since some evaluations can be made with only meager data and information, and thereby suffer the increased likelihood of being invalid.

Measurement is a tool with numerous educational and social functions. Among the most important of these are (1) determining human variability, (2) judging student progress, (3) aiding educational decision making, (4) serving as a common medium for communication, (5) facilitating the whole realm of social and scientific progress.

Mathematics is the common language of measurement. Several scales and basic measurement symbols have been devised for identifying and measuring human differences, and although the technical consideration of statistics is reserved for the next section of this chapter, this preliminary discussion of scales and symbols is a prerequisite to the statistical section.

### Role of Measurement

1. The process of measurement is secondary to that of defining nursing educational objectives. The ends to be achieved must first be formulated. Then measurement procedures can be sought as tools for appraising the extent to which those ends have been achieved.

2. Much of nursing educational and psychological measurement is, and will probably remain, at a relatively low level of precision. We must recognize this fact, using the best procedures available to us, but always treating the resulting score as a tentative hypothesis rather than as an established conclusion.

3. The more elegant procedures of formal tests and measurement must be supplemented by the cruder procedures of informal observation, anecdotal description, and rating if we are to obtain a description of the nursing student that is useful, complete, and comprehensive.

4. No amount of ingenuity in developing improved procedures for measuring and appraising the student will ever eliminate the need to interpret the results from those procedures. Measurement procedures are only tools which provide the data for improved evaluations.

## Scales

Stevens (1951) gives four scale classifications: nominal, ordinal, interval, and ratio. Each of these scales commonly utilizes certain symbols. Those nursing educators who wish a more detailed discussion of the methods of scaling are referred to Stevens or to Torgeson (1965).

*Nominal scales* use a number to designate class, to categorize or to label. Model numbers of cars are an example.

*Ordinal scales* assign numbers on the basis of rank order. Ranking is useful in measurement when the purpose is to determine the relative quality or quantity of a given trait which objects or persons possess. For example, ranking can be used to judge the relative interest of a group of nursing students but the ranks which are assigned apply only within the group and have little relevance for any other group of students. Rank order is often used as a measurement technique when the trait to be measured is intangible and is judged subjectively. The percentile rank technique is a refinement of ranking by which it is possible to determine the percentage of the group which lies below a person within that group. Rank order can be subjected to statistical measurement, including medians, percentiles, and rank order coefficients of correlation.

*Interval scales* have equal units, but the zero point is established and is not absolute; therefore addition of units on the scale is relative to the point at which zero is established. Thus any shift of the arbitrary zero point changes the significance of all numbers as well as their totalled sums. The centigrade thermometer is an example of an interval scale in which an arbitrary or assumed zero has been set at the freezing point of water. With interval scales most of the important statistical calculations are possible.

*Ratio scales* share similarities with the interval scales, but they have an absolute zero established at the point where none of the property represented by the scale exists. All mathematical calculations are possible and meaningful with the ratio scale.

Although the interval and the ratio scales have the greatest number of desirable measurement characteristics, they cannot always be used because of the nature of the behavior being measured. The interval scale is most useful in educational measurement of human characteristics since it is unlikely to find the total absence of any trait.

## Symbols and Definitions

|  |  |
| --- | --- |
| — | Summation sign |
| x, y, z — | Individual score designation |
| f — | Frequency |
| $\overline{X}$, M — | Mean |
| n — | Number in a subgroup |
| N — | Number, total |
| x, d — | Deviation score |
| SD — | Standard deviation (or sigma), S (small s) |
| $S^2, \sigma^2$ — | Variance |

## Scores

**Raw Scores.**   Raw score refers to the weighing of the responses to a test or assessment task by a student. Raw scores are typically the number of right or wrong answers reported in percentages. These raw score percentages are at best weak and difficult to interpret. The scale of measurement found in most educational tests is not an equal unit scale; consequently the measurement information provided by the raw scores is limited. Comparative inferences about student performance based on raw scores are questionable. What is needed, then, owing to the unequal unit scale of measurement of most tests, are ways of transforming raw scores into more meaningful and interpretable data. Statistics is the most reasonable and accurate method of transforming the unequal scale measurements into equal scale measurements. Test results can then be computed and fairly weighted as an index of evaluation.

**Rank-Ordered Scores.**   This refers to the ranking of test scores from highest to lowest, or the reverse, and provides the first step in orderly manipulation of the data to allow better description of test performance. Ranking of scores can provide crude bases for comparison; however, the comparison can be only relative to the set of scores being ranked. The lack of an absolute zero presents a problem. Ranking works best for relatively small sets of scores.

**Intervals of Scores.**   This refers to grouping of scores into intervals, which allows easier management of large numbers of scores. This organized form of data grouping is called a *frequency distribution*. The score column in a frequency distribution must allow for each possible score within the range of scores to be included whether the score exists or not. Here are steps to follow in constructing a frequency distribution:

1. Identify the highest and lowest scores on the test. The distance or spread between these scores is a statistic called the *range*.

2. Determine the number and the size of the intervals to be used in grouping the scores. Odd-numbered interval size (1, 3, 5, and so on) will allow the midpoint of the interval to be a whole number.

The midpoint of the interval 3-7 would be 5. Having the midpoint a whole number does require, however, the lower and upper limits of the interval to be a half number: 2.5 and 7.5 respectively.

> *Example:*
> To determine the number of intervals, select an odd-numbered interval size which, when divided into range of scores, yields from 10 to 15 intervals.
> Use the highest score in the top interval. Set up a table, such as the following one, which will allow easy identification of the *score intervals, tallies, and frequency tallies for each interval.*

*Range of Scores on a Simple Achievement Test*

| Score Intervals | Tallies | Frequency (f) |
|---|---|---|
| 52-56 | / | 1 |
| 47-51 | /// | 3 |
| 42-46 | ////,// | 6 |
| 37-41 | //// | 4 |
| 32-36 | /////,/// | 8 |
| 27-31 | /////,/////,// | 12 |
| 22-26 | /////,//// | 9 |
| 17-21 | /////,// | 7 |
| 12-16 | ///// | 5 |
| 7-11 | // | 2 |
| 2-6 | /// | 3 |
| | | N = 60 |

Range, 56-2
Interval (i) = 5


## The Normal Curve

The normal curve, presented in the chart on page 112, from the Psychological Corporation, illustrates the essential descriptive aspects of the normal curve. Presented directly below the figure are the various percentile equivalents and standard score equivalents plus the stanines.

Examination of the structure of the normal curve indicates that for this theoretical distribution, most of the scores tend to be concentrated at the center of the scale of measurement and gradually taper off to the right and the left from the middle high-point. Since the idealized normal curve is based on the use of an infinite number of scores, the resultant frequency polygon takes on the characteristic of a smooth symmetrical curve, the ends of which theoretically never touch the baseline of the graph. Fifty per cent of the scores lie to the left (toward infinity) of the vertical zero axis which divides the smooth curve into theoretically equal halves, and 50 per cent of the scores lie to the right (toward infinity).

The baseline of the graph is divided into equal divisions marked ±1s, ±2s, ±3s, ±4s from the zero midpoint. The Greek letter sigma is used to designate the standard deviation divisions of the distribution. Each standard deviation is a standard distance along the baseline. Com-

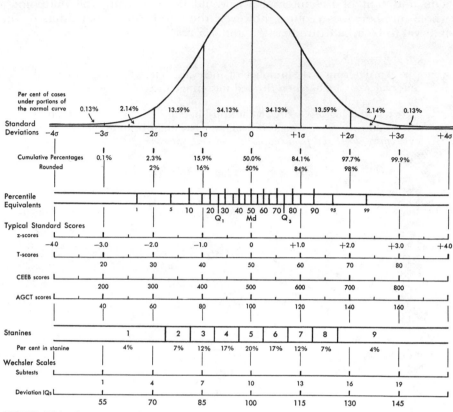

| Per cent of cases under portions of the normal curve | 0.13% | 2.14% | 13.59% | 34.13% | 34.13% | 13.59% | 2.14% | 0.13% |
|---|---|---|---|---|---|---|---|---|
| Standard Deviations | $-4\sigma$ | $-3\sigma$ | $-2\sigma$ | $-1\sigma$ | 0 | $+1\sigma$ | $+2\sigma$ | $+3\sigma$ | $+4\sigma$ |
| Cumulative Percentages | | 0.1% | 2.3% | 15.9% | 50.0% | 84.1% | 97.7% | 99.9% |
| Rounded | | | 2% | 16% | 50% | 84% | 98% | |

Percentile Equivalents
1  5  10  20 30 40 50 60 70 80  90  95  99
$Q_1$  Md  $Q_3$

| Typical Standard Scores z-scores | $-4.0$ | $-3.0$ | $-2.0$ | $-1.0$ | 0 | $+1.0$ | $+2.0$ | $+3.0$ | $+4.0$ |
|---|---|---|---|---|---|---|---|---|---|
| T-scores | | 20 | 30 | 40 | 50 | 60 | 70 | 80 | |
| CEEB scores | | 200 | 300 | 400 | 500 | 600 | 700 | 800 | |
| AGCT scores | | 40 | 60 | 80 | 100 | 120 | 140 | 160 | |

| Stanines | 1 | 2 | 3 | 4 | 5 | 6 | 7 | 8 | 9 |
|---|---|---|---|---|---|---|---|---|---|
| Per cent in stanine | 4% | 7% | 12% | 17% | 20% | 17% | 12% | 7% | 4% |

| Wechsler Scales Subtests | | 1 | 4 | 7 | 10 | 13 | 16 | 19 |
|---|---|---|---|---|---|---|---|---|
| Deviation IQs | | 55 | 70 | 85 | 100 | 115 | 130 | 145 |

NOTE: This chart cannot be used to equate scores on one test to scores on another test. For example, both 600 on the CEEB and 120 on the AGCT are one standard deviation above their respective means, but they do not represent "equal" standings because the scores were obtained from different groups.

putation of the sigma in raw score units will allow the comparative location of a particular score when compared to all the other raw scores. The figure illustrates that with ±3s, 99.72 per cent of all scores are included within the six standard divisions. Most practical needs for comparative identification of raw scores are met by the six divisions, although examination of the curve reveals the ±4s divisions containing 0.26 per cent of the scores.

## Normal Distribution

Any discussion of the distribution of scores brings one to the concept of a normal distribution. Many characteristics are thought to occur with a certain degree of regularity; certain traits are "normally" distributed. Height and weight of individuals vary about a "norm," one for males as well as one for females. In order to aid in the description, inference and prediction of occurrence using statistical theory, the concept of the normal distribution is an important model in educational measurement.

The normal distribution is not an actual distribution of measures, but a theoretical distribution. The theoretical distribution is often represented by a normal probability curve, although it is a mathematical model. Any standard elementary statistical text will carry a detailed account of the origin and structural significance of the probability curve (Ferguson, 1959).

## Percentiles

Percentiles are scores in a distribution below which falls the percentage of scores indicated by the percentile. The median, the middle score or the score where half of the distribution lies above the median and the other half below, is equivalent to the fiftieth percentile. The twenty-fifth and seventy-fifth percentile represent the lower and upper quartiles (Q) of the distribution, where 25 per cent of the scores lie below the twenty-fifth percentile or lower Q and where 75 per cent of the scores lie below the seventy-fifth percentile or upper Q. It may be useful for nursing educators to report test data in percentiles or quartiles to identify comparative rankings of students. Consultation of any elementary statistics text will provide the necessary formulas and the computing steps.

## Percentile Rank

Percentile rank is defined as the percentage of scores in a distribution equal to or lying below a particular score. Percentile rank computations are the reverse of the percentile process. The derivation of the percentile rank begins with an individual score, and the computations determine the percentage of scores which are equal to or lie below that score. The percentile rank process is useful when you want to compare the score of an individual student with scores of others in her group. The formula and directions for computation are presented in any elementary statistics text.

## Measures of Centralness

Measures of centralness or central tendency in a distribution are referred to as averages. There are three widely used averages: median, mode, and arithmetic mean. The *median* is the middle score where half of the distribution lies above the median and the other half below. The *mode* is the score that occurs most frequently in a distribution. The *arithmetic mean* is the quotient derived from dividing the sum of a set of scores by the number of scores (see Tables 1 and 2 for ungrouped data and

grouped data). In a real-life situation, nursing educators will seldom encounter the three measures of central tendency occurring at the same
point in the distribution of test scores. Actual measures or scores seldom
occur in an idealized normal distribution.

## Mean and Standard Deviation

Computation of the mean and standard deviation for ungrouped
scores is illustrated by using the data presented in Table 8-1.

The computation of the mean and standard deviation for grouped
data is essential to the nursing educator who needs to know the average
group score and the degree of distance of each score from the mean.
Using the data in Table 8-2, we can illustrate the computation of the
mean and standard deviation.

Measures of variability such as the standard deviation describe the
way a group of scores differ or vary from each other. The standard deviation of a group of scores is dependent upon the distance of each score
from the mean. The degree of variability or deviance of the scores in the
distribution about the mean determines the way in which standardized

*TABLE 8–1.*

| SCORE | x | $x^2$ |
|---|---|---|
| 25 | 9 | 81 |
| 24 | 8 | 64 |
| 22 | 6 | 36 |
| 22 | 6 | 36 |
| 21 | 5 | 25 |
| 18 | 2 | 4 |
| 17 | 1 | 1 |
| 16 | 0 | 0 |
| 10 | −6 | 36 |
| 9 | −7 | 49 |
| 7 | −9 | 81 |
| 2 | −14 | 196 |
| $\Sigma x = 195$ | | $\Sigma x^2 = 465$ |

N = 12

$$M = \frac{\Sigma x}{N} = \frac{195}{12} = 16.00$$

$$SD = \sqrt{\frac{x^2}{N}} = \sqrt{\frac{465}{12}} = 6.22$$

Where:

$\quad$ M = mean for ungrouped data
$\quad$ SD = standard deviation for ungrouped data

$\quad$ $\Sigma x^2$ = sum of squared deviations from the mean
$\quad$ N = number of cases or scores

*TABLE 8-2.*

| Interval | f | d | fd | fd² |
|----------|---|---|----|----|
| 80-84 | 2 | 6 | 12 | 72 |
| 75-79 | 3 | 5 | 15 | 75 |
| 70-74 | 2 | 4 | 8 | 32 |
| 65-69 | 6 | 3 | 18 | 54 |
| 60-64 | 7 | 2 | 14 | 28 |
| 55-59 | 8 | 1 | 8 | 8 |
| AR = 50-54 | 8 | 0 | 0 | 0 |
| 45-49 | 7 | −1 | −7 | 7 |
| 40-44 | 5 | −2 | −10 | 20 |
| 35-39 | 3 | −3 | −9 | 27 |
| 30-34 | 2 | −4 | −8 | 32 |
| 25-29 | 1 | −5 | −5 | 25 |
| 20-24 | 2 | −6 | −12 | 72 |
| N = 57 | | | $\Sigma$ fd =+24 | $\Sigma$ fd² = 452 |

M = mean for grouped data

$$M = AR + i \left(\frac{fd}{N}\right) = 52 + 5 \left(\frac{24}{57}\right) = 54.11$$

AR = arbitary referrant interval
  i = interval
fd = sum of frequencies times deviances from AR
N = total number of scores
SD − standard deviation for grouped data

$$SD = i \sqrt{\frac{\Sigma fd^2}{N} - \frac{(\Sigma fd)^2}{N}} = 5\sqrt{\frac{452}{57} - \frac{(24)^2}{57}} = 5(2.78) = 13.90$$

$\Sigma$ fd² − sum of the product when multiplying the fd × d = fd²
$(\Sigma fd)^2$ = the squaring of the sum of the f × d = fd

distances about the mean are interpreted. The standard deviation is expressed in raw score units.

Standard Deviations

| −4SD | −3SD | −2SD | −1SD | M | +1SD | +2SD | +3SD | +4SD |
|------|------|------|------|---|------|------|------|------|
| ! | ! | ! | ! | ! | ! | ! | ! | ! |

12.41,   26.31,     40.21, 54.11, 68.01,  81.91,  95.81

The foregoing indicates that the standard deviation of 13.90 means that each standard distance above and below the mean contains 13.90 raw score units of measurement. It appears that the data presented in Table 8-2 show scores which cluster relatively closely about the mean. Large portions of the scores fall within two SDs above and below the mean.

## Standard Scores

Standard deviations can now be used as a basis for computing standard scores. A standard score is the raw score expressed in standard deviation units. Conversion to standard scores provides convenience, comparability, and ease in interpretation of raw score data.

**Z-Scores.** The most basic standard score expresses a raw score in SD units away from the mean. Z-scores show a practical useful range from +3 to −3 SDs. For a Z-score distribution, the mean, M=0, and the SD=1.

**T-Scores.** Commonly thought of as a modified Z-Score, were developed to eliminate the minus and fractional values. For the T-score, the M=50 and the SD=10. The removal of the minus values and the rounding of the fractions to the nearest whole number ease the problem of comparability and consequent interpretation.

### Stanines

This approach is derived from the standard score concept. The stanine plan divides the norm population into nine groups, "standard nine." Except for the top and bottom stanines, groups are spaced in half standard deviation units, where the distribution mean is 5 and the standard deviation is two. Determining the stanine and the percentage of the distribution within each stanine provides increased ease in comparability and interpretation of assessment results.

Ebel (1965) presents a simple method for converting raw scores to stanines for class groups of 20 to 40 students. In its simplest form a stanine scale is a nine-point scale with a mean of five and a standard deviation of two. The percentages of cases included in each stanine are presented here in approximate form:

| STANINE | PER CENT OF CASES | |
|---|---|---|
| 9 | 4 | High |
| 8 | 7 | Above average, 19 per cent |
| 7 | 12 | |
| 6 | 17 | Average, 54 per cent |
| 5 | 20 | |
| 4 | 17 | |
| 3 | 12 | Below Average, 19 per cent |
| 2 | 7 | |
| 1 | 4 | Low |

Stanines also have a distant advantage for punch card data recording, since it takes but one number column on the card to represent a score.

### CORRELATION

Correlation refers to the degree of relationship between two variables. The degree of correlation between two or more variables is expressed by the coefficient of correlation, whose value may extend from +1.00 to 00.00 to −1.00. A coefficient of+1.00 denotes a perfect positive relationship; a coefficient of 00.00 denotes no relationship; and a −1.00 denotes a perfect negative relationship. The correlation coefficient is useful in that it tells us the magnitude and the direction of the relationship. A positive relationship would be indicated by an increase in one variable accompanied by a similar increase in the comparison variable. A negative relationship would be indicated by an increase in one variable accompanied by a decrease in the second variable. Correlation coefficients, although they describe magnitude and direction of the relationship, do not imply that the compared variables have a causal relationship.

The emphasis of the present section on correlation is not to present a detailed analysis and description of correlation, since the writings of many experts in the field of statistics present it much more clearly. The intent is to sensitize the nursing educator to the use of the correlation method in the management and interpretation of measurement data.

Although there are many different techniques for computing correlation coefficients, the techniques most generally used in nursing education measurement questions are the Pearson Product Moment Correlation method and the Spearman Rank Order Correlation Method (see any of the elementary statistics texts for a fuller presentation of the correlation methods).

## STANDARDIZED MEASUREMENT

Usually the comparison of students with other representative groups on a national, regional, state or local basis is made by utilizing standardized tests. The most commonly encountered standardized tests have been developed to measure aptitude, achievement, interest, and personality.

Standardized tests which have gained prominence have been those designed by experts and are a result of many years of preparation, modification, and administration. The gradual refinement of the test instrument will then assess a specific measuring purpose. These tests are prepared to ensure valid, reliable measures which provide accurate norms for student performance evaluation.

### Validity

The validity of a test refers to the degree of accuracy with which it measures what it purports to measure. Validity as a general concept is a matter of degree and is specific to a particular situation.

There are two basic classifications for establishing validity: (1) logical, rational analysis, (2) statistical comparison with an outside criterion.

*Content validity*, arrived at through rational analysis, is concerned primarily with the relation or relevance of the test item to the purpose of the test. Content validity can be specific to a particular situation.

Concurrent and predictive validity are based on statistical evidence. They are both substantiated by comparing the results of a test to an outside criterion. *Predictive validity* is gained through comparison of the test results with a later performance on the criterion, while *concurrent validity* is gained through the comparison of the test results with a current performance on the criterion.

*Construct validity* is the degree to which a test performance can be interpreted to measure certain theorized traits or qualities (constructs). Construct validity tests the underlying theory of the test.

### Reliability

This refers to the degree to which the test measures consistently and accurately what it is supposed to measure. Reliability infers both in terms of repetitive administration and administration over stipulated periods.

The relation between validity and reliability is unclear and needs some clarification. A measuring instrument can provide reliable results without being valid. Conversely, reliability is essential to validity.

The most common methods of obtaining a measure of reliability of an instrument are the test-retest, split half and alternate form comparison. All require statistical comparison resulting in either a reliability coefficient, a coefficient of equivalency, or a coefficient of internal consistency. Reliability can be affected by error, either inherent in the instrument itself or in the administration of the instrument. Because of this variability it is necessary to ensure standardization to calculate a standard error of measurement.

### Norm

Test norms are the statistics which describe the test performance of a highly specified group of persons. The norm provides the range as well as the average performance of the group. Norms allow raw score comparison of an individual test score to larger representative samples of test scores. Norms may be expressed as average performance levels by age or grade classification (age-grade equivalents). Norms may also be expressed as a student's relative position in a comparison group using percentile rank on standard scores.

### Usability

Usability should be a key factor in selection of a test instrument. The ease of administration, scoring, and accuracy in interpretation, plus cost of the test and its administration, scoring, and interpretation, is the main consideration in determining usability of the test.

Factors to be considered in the case of administration are time required, number of subtests, the clarity of the instructions, and simplicity in making responses. Factors related to ease of scoring include ease and speed in hand scoring or machine scoring. Complex testing may require sending the test out to be scored. Ease of interpretation is determined by the degree of complexity in converting raw scores into standard scores and the relative meaning attributed to the standard scores. Interpretation can also be facilitated by ease in identifying and utilizing norm group data for comparison.

## GRADING

Grading is a subjective evaluative process, the composite evaluation of pupil achievement of specified course or performance objectives. The gathering of relevant objective data agreed to as criteria for evaluation by both the nursing educator and student should result in a just and verifiable subjective judgment. The measurement of achievement must be realistically interpreted relative to the philosophy and goals of the instructor, student, and the nursing program.

There should be prior understanding and agreement on the meaning of the grading system used. There should be precise definitions of the meaning for a grade or grade symbol. All behavior thought to be critical in the achievement of the course objective must be examined and defined separately. If, in fact, students are graded or evaluated for attitude, enthusiasm or deportment, these should be so identified and a specific definition of the meaning of a grade presented.

Absolute grading may be related to the theoretical perfect performance, while relative grading may report the comparison of a student's grades to a peer group.

Absolute grading, usually represented in percentages, suffers disadvantages in that it is difficult to determine a total amount of learning that would represent a perfect performance. Also, it is difficult to measure achievement performance with any reasonable accuracy, using percentages.

Absolute grading, however, restated in minimal essential performance, would relate achievement to a degree of mastery. As such, it would eliminate the responsibility of an incompetent performance receiving a high grade simply because it was the best performance out of a set of very poor ones. This grading method would also ensure that all those who performed on a high level would be so identified.

The *pass-fail* absolute grading system, using a tested set of minimal essential critical behaviors which every nurse must be able to demonstrate consistently, may be the most relevant system when it is expected that a nurse is to function in a safe manner. In order to ensure nurse competence in treating patients it may be necessary to establish high standards which have to be exceeded at any point in training or practice. Failure would denote a need for critical review of nurse performance to determine cause for failure. The degree of failure can be judged according to the absolute criteria with some idea of the growth the student must make to pass.

On the other hand, classroom or subject matter achievement may be better suited to a relative grading system. In this situation *letter grades* appear to be more advantageous to the student. There is a problem, however, in the use of a relative grading system due to the difficulty in accurately defining what is typical achievement for a peer group. Most relative grading systems are referred to the normal curve which assumes achievement performance to be normally distributed. This assumption may be indefensable in that the nursing students may represent a more homogeneous group. Selection and performance criteria prior to admission to nursing may significantly increase the performance homogeneity of the student nurses so there is little variability and a consequent non-normally distributed group.

The most difficult area of student performance to evaluate would be in the clinical situation. Although nursing educators use minimal essential levels of performance, it is still difficult to establish valid and reliable criteria for judging "safe" nursing practice. In addition is the need to examine different rates of professional growth among the students. How many mistakes do you allow the student to make? How long is she allowed to overcome the errors in nursing judgment and performance? Counseling and guidance could be valuable service to the student nurse who is faced with failure or near success. Counseling could help the student reexamine her abilities and concerns about failure.

A grade or any other evaluative report is of no value unless the student feels that the grade truly represents actual achievement and specifies areas where there is failure. Good reporting of student status and progress would allow the nurse-counselor to respond more accurately to the student nurse's needs.

Chapter 9

# Construction of Classroom Tests

In Chapter 8 we discussed the overall concept of evaluation in nursing education. We included an analysis of behavioral objectives, basic measurement principles, and grading. All evaluation procedures, however, are merely tools or means to an end, the end in this case being a systematic, fair, and objective assessment of students' knowledge, abilities, and understanding. In this chapter we shall apply these measurement principles to the construction of classroom tests. This will include the various kinds of tests and examinations, such as essay and objective and oral examinations, In the next chapter we shall apply the same principles to the area of clinical evaluation.

## FRAME OF REFERENCE FOR TEST CONSTRUCTION

Any test is a sample of a student's knowledge and behavior. From this sample, inferences can be made about the student's ability, capacity, character, achievement, or whatever dimension that is purportedly related to the test results. Thus on the basis of one or more samples, inferences about the student's behavior in non-test situations can be made. A test is a sample of a student's behavior on the assumption that the behavior demonstrated in the test situation is indicative of behavior in nontest situations, e.g. ability to apply knowledge in the clinical area.

In constructing a test or any evaluation procedure, we must begin by deciding what kinds of decisions we want to make. What do we need to know about this student? What do we want to be able to say about this student after we have obtained a sample of her behavior? In brief, evaluation is always for a purpose, and that purpose should be clearly stated so that we may select appropriate samples of behavior, and be able to make appropriate judgments based on sound principles.

In trying to answer the foregoing questions, we are likely to experience some difficulty, for it is not always easy to define the properties of behavior in which we are interested. Such difficulties are in part related to the fact that when we attempt to measure psychological traits, such as sensitivity to the needs of another person, we can measure such traits only indirectly in terms of their manifestations in the overt behavior of individuals. Nevertheless, despite the inherent difficulty involved in defining the traits to be measured, or in specifying the kinds of decisions to be made, it is still an essential part of assessment in nursing education.

After we have defined what we want to evaluate, then we select appropriate situations for calling forth the behavior, devise some method for obtaining a record of the behavior, and develop some procedure for summarizing or evaluating the behavior as recorded. In some cases the behavior can be assessed only in the clinical area. At this point, however, we are primarily concerned with the kinds of knowledge and behavior that can be readily assessed in the classroom. In deciding on the procedures to be followed, we really need to be concerned with the answers to several basic questions:

1. What decisions do I want the test results to help me to make? For example, how may I best measure the student's ability to function at least at a minimal level of competency for safe nursing care?

2. What data or behavioral samples do I need in order to make these decisions? What data can be collected in the classroom, and what must be held for the clinical area?

Let us take a look at the first question. What decisions do I want the test results to help me to make? Note that we are not asking the test itself to make decisions. We are asking for assistance in making decisions. In answering this question, it is helpful to raise a number of subordinate questions. Do I want the test results to help me to determine a fair grade for each student based on her overall performance? Do I want the test results to help me determine the student's pattern of strengths and weaknesses?

When these subordinate questions have been asked and answered, a second basic question must then be asked. What data or behavioral samples do I need in order to make these decisions? The subordinate questions to be considered are these: What kinds of items, questions or problems shall I use? Shall I permit the students to use reference materials? Do I need questions that vary in levels and range of difficulty? The following provides a working model for the frame of reference which has been introduced here (Furst, 1958).

*Frame of Reference Work Sheet*

| What decisions do I want the test results to help me make? | What data do I need in order to make these decisions? |
| --- | --- |
| 1. We want to determine a fair grade for each student based on overall performance | A total score based on a representative sampling of the course |
| 2. We want to be able to tell a student her pattern of strength and weakness<br><br>　a. The degree to which she has acquired the basic information<br>　b. The degree to which she can choose the right course of action | Part scores for each type of outcome<br>Each part score must show the relative level of accomplishment so that part scores may be compared |

c. The degree to which she can support her choices by citing appropriate principles

| | |
|---|---|
| 3. We want to be able to identify students who have acquired a good fund of information, but have not developed much facility in applying it | A scatter diagram relating scores from 2a above with scores on a composite of b and c would be helpful. Also clinical evaluation tools are useful here |
| 4. We want to be able to identify students who are good at choosing the correct course of action, but are unable to rationalize their choices | An examination of the part scores corresponding to a and b under 2 above |
| 5. We want to be able to determine whether there is a high correlation between scores on information and scores on application | Similar to the data needed for 3 above. A coefficient would give a summary index of the degree of relationship |
| 6. We want to be able to decide where our instruction has been effective and where it needs improvement | All the above would be helpful. It would also be desirable to get item analysis data showing the proportion of students who have been successful on the various items of the test |

## SOME GENERAL CONSIDERATIONS

After the kinds of decisions to be made are determined, and the data needed for making these decisions have been specified, then the test must be constructed. The items must be written and selected, and the length of the test must be determined; the physical make-up of the test, and the scoring system are other problems which remain and must be resolved. It should be emphasized from the very beginning that written tests are but one tool of measurement: others include oral tests, clinical or situational tests, anecdotal records, systematic observation and ratings, sociometric devices, and so forth.

In writing test items the faculty member is selecting and constructing the task which will secure the data which is needed in order for the decision to be made. The most widely used procedure for the construction of test items involves the writing of items for each topic and subtopic presented in the course outline or in the text outline. The instructor looks at the topic, decides on the sort of question she wishes to write to measure whether the student has mastered facts or concepts, and then writes the item. When this is done, topics which are of the greatest importance should have more items associated with them.

A simple procedure that can be followed in collecting test items is always to carry some 3 by 5 or 5 by 8 cards with you. When you read the text or other reading assignments, jot down questions or test items which may be used later. In other words, collect assessment material while you collect teaching material. When you get an idea, write the item down. Do not be concerned with the actual writing at this point, for when the items are selected, careful editing will correct the deficiencies of earlier items. When the time comes for selecting items for the test, the instructor has a pool of items from which to choose. Through the years the test item file is increased and modified as new items come to mind and old ones are re-evaluated and modified in the light of experience.

Some additional guidelines that should be considered are the following:

1. Use as many items as possible that require the student to apply learning or to function at higher cognitive levels.

2. Include items at different levels of difficulty. This tends to produce a significant range of scores and facilitates decision making.

3. Make each item realistic and practical. One way to do this is to identify desired responses and then to construct items which will elicit these responses.

4. Underline crucial words to increase the readability of test items.

5. Word questions so that the correct answers require a knowledge of the subject.

6. Avoid trick or "catch" questions.

7. Keep the reading difficulty of the test items low.

8. Do not lift a statement verbatim from the text.

9. If an item is based on opinion or an authority, state whose.

10. Avoid ambiguity of statement and meaning.

11. Avoid items dealing with trivia.

12. Prepare a scoring key with correct answers.

13. Give clear directions on what the student is expected to do.

## THE OBJECTIVE EXAMINATION

The objective examination includes such questions as multiple choice, true-false, matching, classification, identification, listing, completion, and single answer. It has certain unique and essential features, as follows:

1. The test is completely structured.

2. Except for single-answer and completion items, the student selects the correct answer from among a limited number of alternatives.

3. The sample of items is large.

4. Each item has a clearly predetermined answer.

5. The test is relatively free of opportunities to bluff.

6. Anyone can score the tests with a scoring key.

7. The test is time-consuming to prepare, but is quick to score.

### Completion Test Items

A *single-answer item* requires the student to find or recall one item of information. It is usually reserved for situations in which the student must remember specific information, for it measures only memory. It can be used, however, to familiarize the student in the use of reference materials by requiring her to find specific items in the material. When constructed, it should imply that there is only one correct answer, and it should require the correct answer to be given in either a single word or in a concise statement.

An example of the single answer type item is as follows:

Directions: Each of the questions listed below has but one correct answer. Express your answer as briefly and concisely as possible. The value of each test item is 3 points.

1. When aphasia occurs, which body system has probably been impaired?

_____

2. Cardiology is a subspecialty of what branch of medicine? _____

_____

The simple *completion-type item* is similar to the single-answer type of question in that it requires the student to recall and supply certain definite and exact information. It consists of incomplete statements in which one or more key words have been omitted. The words, when recalled and placed in appropriate blanks, make the statement complete, meaningful, and true. The main characteristics of completion test items are as follows:

1. The simple completion item can be used to test student ability to recall specific facts; it demands accurate information.

2. It can be used effectively to sample a wide range of subject matter.

3. It can be used in paragraph form to test continuous thought within a specific area of subject matter.

4. It can be used to discriminate effectively.

5. Used indiscriminately, it tends to measure verbal facility and memorizing of facts rather than application.

6. It has the disadvantage of being difficult to make entirely objective.

Some samples of completion test items follow:

Directions: Complete the meaning of each statement by writing the correct word or phrase in each blank. The value of each test item is 5 points.
1. Groups of more or less similar cells form body _____
2. From the right side of the heart, blood is routed to the _____
3. Most of the digestion of food takes place in the _____
4. Two factors that cause a temporary rise in the blood pressure are _____
_____ and _____

There are certain guidelines to follow in the construction of completion test items. These are:

1. Write out a number of factual and important statements based on the instruction. Do not copy statements directly from the text studied by students.

2. Substitute blanks for key words. Omit no more than three words in a sentence. A short sentence with only one word omitted is preferable.

3. Reword each statement, if necessary, so that it will remain incomplete until the correct word or phrase is inserted. Make all blanks the same length regardless of the length of the omitted word(s). Place the blanks near the end or at least past the middle of the sentence.

4. If possible, construct the item so that there can be only one correct response.

5. Do not omit verbs. Avoid being too brief. Make the statement complete enough so that there is no doubt as to its meaning.

6. Avoid indefinite or "open" completion items.

7. If the problem requires a numerical answer, indicate the units in which it is to be expressed.

8. Avoid "a" or "an" immediately before a blank.

### Multiple-Choice Items

The multiple-choice item consists of two parts. The first part, usually referred to as the problem, either asks a question or takes the form of an incomplete statement. It serves as the stem for the second part, which consists of several alternatives that are possible answers to the question presented, or are possible completions of the incomplete statement. One alternative is either the clearly best one or the only correct answer. The other alternatives are plausible but incorrect answers.

The main characteristics of multiple choice items are as follows:

1. The scoring of the multiple-choice item is objective.

2. Its design can be varied to suit many kinds of subject matter and to measure various kinds of achievement.

3. It can be designed to present problems involving reasoning and judgment based on knowledge. Such items require the student to use her knowledge rather than merely her memory for facts.

4. It can measure ability to use reasoning, form judgments, and apply learning. It can also measure recognition, which has a larger scope than recall.

5. Although it tests the student's recognition of the correct answer from among a series of possible answers, it does not indicate with certainty whether the student would have recalled the correct answer without any hints.

6. It cannot test the student's ability to organize and present her knowledge in her own language, which may be an important factor in the educational outcome desired.

An example of a multiple-choice item with a statement to be completed is as follows:

> Directions: Each of the incomplete statements or questions which are given below is followed by several possible answers. Select the *best* answer for each test item. Indicate your answer by circling the letter corresponding to the response chosen. The value of each test item is 1 point.

1. Health may be defined as
   a. Absence from disease
   b. Not being ill very often
   c. A sense of well-being
   d. Immunity to disease

The following is an example of a multiple-choice item that has a question to be answered:

1. What is the best definition of otosclerosis?
   a. An acute condition with temporary loss of hearing
   b. An impairment due to injury of the auditory nerve with permanent deafness
   c. A progressive condition that results from hardening of the ossicles of the middle ear
   d. A condition resulting from a perforation of the eardrum

There are several guidelines to use in constructing multiple-choice items. These are as follows:

1. Include at least four, but not more than five, alternative or possible responses.

2. List possible responses in a column. This makes them easier to read and less confusing to answer.

3. When the stem is an incomplete statement, place the blank for the correct choice of alternatives at the end of the statement. This provides better continuity when the item is read. If answers are to be written on the test paper itself, then the answer spaces should be brought out to the left or right of the question and arranged in a column for quick and simple scoring.

4. The item should test only one idea and should contain only material relevant to its solution. Avoid questions on trivial details, and questions that can be answered solely on the basis of intelligence or general knowledge.

5. Omit responses that are obviously wrong. Word all responses in such a manner that the student must know the subject matter to select the correct answer from the incorrect but fairly plausible answers.

6. When a negative item is used, emphasize the negative word or phrase. It can be underlined, capitalized or italicized.

7. Avoid clues to the correct answer. Avoid, for example, "a" or "an" as the final word in the stem unless all alternatives begin with a consonant or all begin with a vowel. Scatter the position of the correct answers and avoid any pattern of placing them.

8. When words or phrases are common to all alternatives, place them in the stem.

9. When several stems have the same alternatives, consider presenting the subject matter as a matching-test item instead.

10. The stem should clearly formulate a problem. Don't load the stem with irrelevant material.

11. Be sure that there is only one correct or clearly best answer.

12. Avoid cues from the length of the alternative. The correct answer tends to be longer.

## True-False or Alternative-Answer Items

The true-false item consists of a simple statement to be marked true or false. The main characteristics of this kind of item are as follows:

1. The true-false item can be made a factual question or a thought that requires reasoning.

2. It can be used as an instructional test item to promote interest and to introduce points for discussion.

3. It can sample effectively a wide range of subject matter.

4. It has the disadvantage of being difficult to construct, for it is difficult to make a statement completely true or false without making the correct response apparent.

5. Since there are only two alternative answers for this sort of item, it encourages guessing. Half of the questions might be answered correctly without any knowledge of the subject.

6. A large number of true and false items are required to discriminate between the good and the weak students.

7. Its scoring is objective and easy.

Some examples of true-false items are as follows:

Directions: Listed below are a number of statements; some are true and some are false. If any part of a statement is false, the entire statement is false. Make your decision by circling T if the item is true, and F if the item is false. The value for each test item is 1 point.

T F    1. Hypothermia refers to lowering of the body temperature.
T F    2. In most cases the human body rejects tissue from another body.
T F    3. Damage to the radial nerve is likely to result from the prolonged use of crutches if the crutches are too heavy.
T F    4. Insulin, cortisone, and ACTH are all hormone drugs.

There are several guidelines to follow in constructing true-false items. These are as follows:

1. Prepare approximately the same number of true statements as false statements. Mix them thoroughly, but not in any set pattern.

2. Avoid cues from the length of the statement. Do not make the true statements consistently longer than the false statements.

3. Require application of things learned in as many items as possible.

4. Avoid negatives, double negatives, and involved statements.

5. Avoid specific determiners. Statements with "all," "only," "none," "never," and "always" are usually false. Statements with the words "generally" and "usually" have a tendency to be true.

6. Avoid ambiguous indefinite terms of degree or amount. For example, what does "frequently" mean?

7. Avoid items that include more than one idea, especially if one is true and the other is false.

8. Avoid the exact language of the textbook.

9. Avoid trick questions or trivia.

10. Require the simplest possible method of indicating the correct response. For example, circle the T or F, mark the answer sheet, place + for true and 0 for false in the space provided.

## Matching-Test Items

The matching type of test item consists of two lists of related-words, phrases, clauses or symbols. The student is required to match or pair each item in one list with the one item in the other list to which it is most closely related. The main characteristics of matching test items are as follows:

1. The matching type of test item is especially valuable for measuring student ability to recognize relationships and make associations.

2. It is highly reliable, discriminating, and objective.

3. It can be used in many relationships, such as matching terms with definitions, symbols with names, questions with answers, cause with effect, parts with functions, procedures with operations, and principles with situations in which the principles apply.

4. It has the disadvantage of being a poor measure of interpretation and understanding.

5. It is less desirable than the multiple-choice item for measuring judgments and applications of things taught.

A sample of a matching-test item is as follows:

Directions: In the two columns below are listed the names of famous scientists and their scientific contributions. The names in Column I are identified by numbers; those in Column II by letters. The task is to match or pair each number in Column I with the appropriate letter in Column II. Each letter in Column II may be selected only once. Place the appropriate letter in the space provided by each number. The value for each test item is 1 point.

|  Column I | Column II |
|---|---|
| ( ) 1. Banting, Macleod, and Best | a. Discovery of oral poliomyelitis vaccine |
| ( ) 2. Marie and Pierre Curie | b. Discovery of radium |
| ( ) 3. Fleming | c. Discovery of insulin |
| ( ) 4. Koch | d. Discovery of heart catheterization |
| ( ) 5. Lister | e. Discovery of X-ray |
| ( ) 6. Pasteur | f. Pioneer in antiseptic methods |
| ( ) 7. Roentgen | g. Pioneer work in bacteriology in France |
|  | h. Pioneer work in bacteriology in Germany |
|  | i. Discovery of penicillin |
|  | j. Introduction of more humane methods of surgery in the 1500's |

Some guidelines to be used in constructing matching-test items are as follows:

1. Require at least 5 and not more than 12 responses, there should

be at least 3 extra items from which responses may be chosen, unless a response may be used more than once.

2. Place the column containing the longer phrases or clauses on the right side of the page.

3. State in the directions the area to which the things listed apply. List nothing in either column that is not relevant to the subject.

4. Response options should be listed in a logical order, if one exists, e.g. dates.

5. Directions should clearly indicate whether an answer may be used more than once.

6. All items should be on the same page.

## Classification-Test Items

The classification-test item is another form of the matching-test item. It requires the student to classify several terms, phrases or clauses in terms of definite categories. It is used instead of the matching-test item when several things listed in an exercise bear a definite relationship to other things listed. The classification-test item has essentially the same characteristics as the matching-test item; the same rules should be used in constructing both types.

An example of a classification test item is the following:

Directions:  In the two columns below are listed some body systems and some of the principal impairments associated with these systems. The impairments, identified by numbers, appear in Column I. The systems, identified by letters, appear in Column II. The task is to classify the items in Column I under the items in Column II. Place the appropriate letter in the space provided by each number. The value of each test item is 2 points.

| Column I | Column II |
|---|---|
| (  )  1. Prostatitis | a. Musculoskeletal |
| (  )  2. Diverticula | b. Cardiovascular |
| (  )  3. Paraplegia | c. Genitourinary |
| (  )  4. Hemorrhoids | d. Gastrointestinal |
| (  )  5. Arteriosclerosis | e. Respiratory |
| (  )  6. Emphysema | f. Hemic-lymphatic |
| (  )  7. Nephritis | g. Nervous |
| (  )  8. Hepatitis | h. Endocrine |
| (  )  9. Phlebitis | |
| (  ) 10. Ankylosis | |
| (  ) 11. Apoplexy | |
| (  ) 12. Scoliosis | |
| (  ) 13. Myxedema | |
| (  ) 14. Coronary infarct | |
| (  ) 15. Hodgkin's disease | |

## Identification-Test Items

The identification-type test item is used to measure student ability to recall and give the proper names of such things as symbols, specific parts, mechanical units, or instruments. The main characteristics of identification test items are as follows:

1. The identification-test item can be substituted for the matching item when it is desired to have students recall and indicate the proper names of tools, symbols, instruments or specific parts.

2. It can measure the application of knowledge, as in detecting errors in a drawing.

Several examples of identification-test items are given below:

Directions: In the corresponding numbered blanks to the right of the drawing, write the name of the part represented by each number. The value of each test item is 1 point.

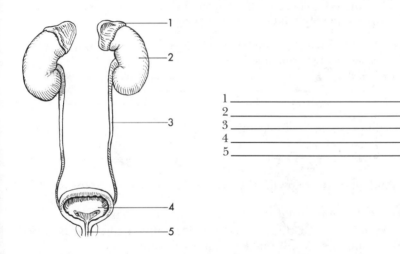

1 _____
2 _____
3 _____
4 _____
5 _____

Directions: In the corresponding numbered blanks to the right of the common abbreviations shown below, write the word or phrase for which the abbreviation stands. The value for each item is 1 point.

1. q.i.d.          1._____
2. ss              2._____
3. o.m.            3._____
4. Stat.           4._____

There are several guidelines to follow in the construction of identification test items. These are as follows:

1. Make all drawings clear.

2. Check that only one definite answer is possible.

3. Make sure that the lines indicating the parts to be named terminate at the proper places.

## Listings or Enumeration-Test Items

The listing or enumeration-test item requires the student to supply a list of terms, or factors, that have been taught. Students may or may not be required to list the items in a particular order. Some characteristics of these items are as follows:

1. The listing type of item measures the degree of recall of specific points of information.

2. It reduces the possibility of guessing the right answer.

3. It allows some freedom of expression.

4. It places too much emphasis upon memorizing facts and details.

5. It tends to become somewhat objective.

6. It cannot measure readily the student's ability to use or to interpret information.

Some examples of listing or enumeration test-items are as follows:

Directions: Read each item carefully. Follow the directions given with each. The value of each test item is 5 points.

In the spaces provided below, list the symptoms usually associated with pneumonia.

1._____   5._____
2._____   6._____
3._____   7._____
4._____

List two causes of hepatitis.

1._____
2._____

Several guidelines to follow in the construction of such items are the following:

1. Design each item so that it will call for specific facts.

2. Make sure that each thing listed involves only a few words. Lists of long complex statements will make scoring subjective.

3. Restrict the question so that no more than 6 to 8 things are required to be listed in the answer.

4. Do not use a question unless the possible responses are limited and specific.

## THE CORRECTION FOR GUESSING

Occasionally, faculty members become concerned over the fact that students seem to be guessing at the right answer on objective test items rather than really knowing the correct answer. One way of handling this problem is to apply the correction for guessing formula. For true-false tests, the formula is simply:

$R - W$ = final score
$R$ = the number of items correct
$W$ = the number of items incorrect

For multiple choice questions, the formula is:

$$R - \frac{W}{N-1}$$

R = the number of items correct
W = the number of items incorrect
N = the number of possible choices on each question

The correction for guessing is usually used in true-false examinations which have less than 50 items or on multiple-choice questions with only three choices. The formula should never be used without warning the students in advance. This can be done by explaining the correction for guessing and the rationale for its use. In addition, the test directions should include a statement approximating the following: Omit those items that you can answer only by pure guess.

## ITEM ANALYSIS

An important step in the evaluation of objective tests is the item analysis. The item analysis gives a check on the internal validity of the test through a comparison of the students' performance on each test item against their total test scores. The item analysis consists in the determination of the percentage of students in the high test group and the percentage in the low test group who answered each item correctly. It is designed to provide information about the difficulty level of each item and about the ability of each item to discriminate between good and poor students. Items on which a higher percentage of good students than poor students answer correctly show positive discrimination. Negative discrimination occurs when the poor students answer an item correctly more frequently than the good students. Items which show negative discrimination are usually discarded.

Item analysis performed on a test that has been constructed carelessly will provide little if any discrimination. For best results there should be at least 100 test papers from which to select those to be item-analyzed. The following procedure describes the method to be followed for determining the quality and difficulty of the test items.

1. Select the top 30 per cent and the bottom 30 per cent of the papers.

2. Working with one group at a time, arrange the papers on a large table so that they overlap with only the response column on each paper visible.

3. Count the number of correct responses on each item, convert to percentages, and enter the result on a record sheet. For example, if 16 out of 20 in one group answered the item correctly, 80 per cent should be entered on the record sheet for that item.

4. After the correct responses on all items have been counted for both the high and low groups, the power of the item can be determined from the percentage in both groups who responded correctly. Thus,

when 28 of the 40 students have answered an item correctly, the ease index is 70 per cent, or, conversely, the index of difficulty is 30 per cent.

5. Calculate the item discrimination with the following formula:

$$D = \frac{U - L}{N}$$

U = number of students in upper group answering item correctly
L = number of students in lower group answering item correctly
N = number of students in each group

The discrimination index ranges from +1 to −1, but only items which show positive indices should be retained. A discrimination index above +0.40 is desirable.

Of course this whole process is made considerably simpler if computer manipulation of the items is performed. Attention should also be paid to the incorrect responses on each item. If a response on an item draws no students, then it is apparently too obvious a distractor and should be replaced. For example, on a multiple-choice item with four possible responses, if no one in the class selects response 3, then it is a worthless distractor and should be replaced. Although the process of item analysis takes time, it is necessary to ensure continuing improvement of the objective tests given in the classroom.

## ESSAY EXAMINATIONS

In the essay type of examination the student is required to make a comparison, write a description, or explain some aspect of the subject she is studying. There are certain essential characteristics of the essay examination.

1. The student organizes her own answers with a minimum of restraint. The question requires the student to produce rather than merely to recognize the answers. It minimizes the possibility of getting the answers by blind guessing or by using little cues to outguess the test maker.

2. The student uses her own words and her own handwriting. This places a premium upon verbal fluency and skill of expression. Students also are frequently penalized for poor handwriting.

3. The student answers a small number of questions. If we ask what the student knows and has studied, fine; otherwise, she does poorly.

4. The student produces answers with all degrees of completeness and accuracy As a result, the examinations are time-consuming to correct, and grading tends to be highly subjective.

5. The examination can be prepared rapidly.

The advantages claimed for the essay type of examination are as follows:

1. It tests ability to understand, interpret, reason, discriminate, and generalize.

2. It tests ability to use and apply what has been learned.

3. It measures ability to recall, evaluate, select, and organize material systematically.

4. It tests accuracy in expression and coherence in composition.

5. Nearly every question allows the student some range of choice.

6. It is acceptable in almost any situation; it is easy to make and administer.

Some of the common objections to the essay examination are as follows:

1. Because the grading is subjective and may be easily influenced by irrelevant matters such as the instructor's personal attitudes and prejudices, it is not exactly fair to the student.

2. Because of the length of time required for answering the questions, only a few can be asked, and thus the test can cover only a limited range of material.

3. It is difficult to score because the questions are vague.

4. Because it is almost impossible to set up exact and uniform norms and standards, it is difficult to interpret the scores or grades made.

5. Its use often results in negative student attitudes because of the difficulties attendant on subjective scoring.

6. Because it does not require exact information, it is easy for the examinee to bluff and pad her answers.

7. It is uninteresting to both the instructor and the student because it lacks variety in the kinds of questions asked.

There are certain times when it is definitely more desirable to administer an essay examination than an objective test. These include the following reasons:

1. When the class is small
2. When the time to prepare the test is limited
3. When you wish to test abilities to select, relate, and organize, to create essentially new patterns, and to use language to express one's ideas
4. Not when the reproduction of factual information is desired.

Several examples of essay questions used in nursing education are as follows:

Directions: For each set of concepts listed below, indicate the way in which they are different. The value of each item is 25 points.
1. Physical medicine, physical therapy, and occupational therapy
2. Congenital, neoplastic, traumatic, and metabolic
3. Multiple sclerosis and arthritis
Directions: Criticize each of the following statements. The value of each item is 20 points.
1. "Stress is the chief cause of the large number of heart attacks."
2. "Psychotherapy is the treatment of choice in psychosomatic illness."
Directions: Give short answers to the following questions. The value of each item is 10 points.
1. Why is the blood pressure of patients with CVA's measured at frequent and regular intervals?
2. Why are certain persons who frequently are emotionally upset more prone to colitis, constipation, and diarrhea?

3. Under what circumstances may catheterization be ordered by a physician?

There are certain guidelines to follow in the construction of essay examinations which will greatly improve their effectiveness. These are as follows:

1. Call for specific answers. Word the item so that the student has an outline she can follow in formulating her response. Make certain that the points scored are apparent. Avoid general questions that encourage the windbag or that elicit different and difficult-to-score answers from each student.

2. Replace the one long general question with one or more of a series of shorter, more specific ones.

3. If the questions cover material of different importance, the scoring weight for each question should reflect its importance and be clearly communicated to the student in advance.

4. Each student should be required to answer the same questions. Giving students a choice of questions reduces the common base on which all students may be compared.

5. Design the essay item in a way to require students to:

*Compare*—Give similarities and differences. Set the items side by side and show their similarities or resemblances. A two-column listing of these is a good form of answer.

*Contrast*—Stress the differences or dissimilarities.

*Define*—Give the category, or a short, clear, and accurate statement. Don't give illustrations unless absolutely necessary.

*Criticize*—Point out errors or weaknesses, or find fault with the item.

*Explain*—Tell and show how. In order to give a clear picture, often an illustration will help. *Explain why* indicates offering reasons; *explain how* indicates using a logical sequence.

*Illustrate*—Provide examples. Give a good, clear, and pertinent example, instance or case. Omit definitions.

*List*—Write only a series of items. Don't discuss or illustrate.

*Outline*—Give the main points only, without details, and with little or no discussion. Using an accepted form of outline will help to show the relative importance and relationships of items.

*Prove*—Give evidence. List the arguments in favor of the item. Sometimes a similar list of arguments against the objections to this item will be helpful.

*State*—Express ideas briefly and clearly. Don't discuss in detail or illustrate.

*Summarize*—In a short and concise manner, sum up the main fact expected in the response.

There are also several guidelines which will improve the objectivity of scoring an essay examination. These are as follows:

1. Decide in advance what factors are to be measured. If more than one distinct quality is to be appraised, make separate evaluations of each, e.g. facts, organization, process.

2. Prepare a model answer in advance, showing what points are desired and the credit to be allowed for each.

3. Read all the answers to one question before going on to the next.

4. Grade the papers as nearly anonymously as possible.

5. Greater reliability can be obtained by averaging independent ratings.

6. Examinations should always be scored by the one who makes out the questions.

Several variations of the essay examination are sometimes used which are subject to the same guidelines as those stated above. The first of these is the *take-home* or *out-of-class* examination. This has the advantage of allowing the student unlimited time to prepare, organize, and submit the best answers she can. It has the disadvantage at times of placing the instructor in the position of wondering who wrote the responses. It is an excellent technique to use when you are primarily interested in the student's ability to search out the appropriate information to support a carefully thought-out position.

A second variation is the *open-book examination.* This is useful when the student needs access to tables, formulas or other reference information that would be unreasonable to memorize and useless in terms of future practice.

A third variation is the *master list* or *study questions.* In this technique, students are given a comprehensive list of questions that thoroughly cover all the material in the unit or course. They are told that the examination will be made up of questions drawn from the list. This has the advantage of forcing students to study in a comprehensive fashion, and ensuring that they recognize the important areas to be emphasized.

The final variation sometimes used is the *oral examination.* This has relatively little practical value in the classroom. It has poor validity and reliability. It leaves no record of the student's work, is highly vulnerable to subjectivity and bias, and, finally, is too time-consuming.

## SITUATION OR PROBLEM-SOLVING EXAMINATIONS

The presentation of various questions through the use of situations or problems is usually referred to as a situation-type or problem-solving type of examination. Strictly speaking, it is not a form of test item, for the situation or problem may be followed by essay, listing, or any other kind of test item. The characteristics of a situation-type test are as follows:

1. The test is one of the most valuable methods for measuring a student's ability to apply things she has previously learned.

2. It can be varied or adapted to various kinds of subject matter.

3. It is sometimes difficult to make objective.

4. Although highly valid, it must be carefully constructed and scored.

5. It does not require that test items be grouped according to type.

Several examples of the situation or problem-solving type of question would be the following:

When you are about to insert the needle for an injection, Mr. W. tenses his muscles. What action should you take? You are told by Mr. W. that the doctor has advised him that it is dangerous for him to get angry. Mr. W. says, "I've got plenty to rile me. How can I keep from getting angry?" How would you answer him? Why?

Directions: In the following section, questions are centered in real patient situations. In each case select the one best answer and place the corresponding number in the space following the number of the question. The value of each item is 2 points.

Mr. W., 22 years old, is a patient in the medical unit of a general hospital. His diagnosis is sclerosing nephritis. His blood pressure is 210/150. He has generalized edema and shortness of breath. His urine output is scanty. The doctor has ordered (1) complete bed rest; (2) low-salt, moderate-protein, high-vitamin diet; (3) limitation of fluids to 1000 cc. daily; (4) ammonium chloride gr.× t.i.d.; (5) mercuhydrin 1 cc. I.M. q.d.× 3 days.

1. You recall that nephritis is a condition in which there is an involvement of the
   a. Gallbladder  1._____
   b. Urinary bladder
   c. Nephrons
   d. Kidneys
   e. Glomeruli
2. Mr. W's urine contains albumin. this means that     2._____
   a. Bits of tissue are being excreted from the damaged kidneys
   b. There is a sloughing away of the walls of the bladder
   c. There is an abnormal amount of sugar in the urine
   d. His condition is improving
   e. None of the above
3. One of the drugs that Mr. W. receives is a diuretic which
   a. Increases the flow of urine
   b. Increases his blood pressure
   c. Increases the absorption of sodium chloride
   d. Decreases thirst
   e. All of the above
4. To relieve Mr. W's dyspnea, the best nursing measure would be to
   a. Place Mr. W. in a prone position
   b. Encourage him to eat all the food served him
   c. Raise the head of his bed to a 45 ° angle
   d. Massage gently his swollen ankles and feet
   e. None of the above

In the construction of situation-type tests, the following guidelines should prove helpful:

1. Make the item as specific as possible.
2. Make it require the student to solve a problem.
3. Include directions for recording the response in the directions to fit all situations.
4. State the problems or describe the situation clearly and concisely. Use sketches if possible. Avoid extraneous material.
5. Avoid basing the solution to one problem on the response to another.

## OTHER FACTORS TO BE CONSIDERED IN TEST CONSTRUCTION

There are several other factors in addition to those previously discussed that must be taken into consideration in the construction of tests. These factors pertain to the initial assembling of the test, the directions to the student, and to the use of separate answer sheets. With respect to the task of assembling the test, the following recommendations may be helpful.

1. Introduce the test by a full identification and description. In the introduction give complete instructions for taking the test, list the references and aids the student may use, if any, and explain the recording of answers. These instructions should always be given even if it may be assumed that the student has had experience with similar tests.

2. Group items by types (e.g. true-false, multiple choice).

3. Arrange items within each type so that related material appears together.

4. Exclude any item that supplies, or depends upon, the answer to another.

5. Arrange the items so that the correct answers will form a random pattern.

6. Base the joint value of each test item on the amount of achievement it measures.

In addition to the directions contained in the introduction to the test, there are two other sets of directions to be given the student. The first revolves around the general orientation to testing given all students. They should be taught in advance how to take tests, and told in advance exactly what sort of test will be given each time. This last point is a necessary one, for students study differently for different kinds of tests. The second deals with the specific directions for each kind of test item. Such directions should state clearly and concisely what students are required to do, how to indicate the answers, and where the answer is to be placed. Examples are part of the directions and should be given when necessary.

As for the use of answer sheets, these may be provided for objective-type examinations. The use of answer sheets eliminates the necessity of turning pages when marking the test, decreases the probability of errors in scoring, and permits the use of a template for scoring.

After each test it is extremely desirable to go over the test with the students question by question. In so doing, the test becomes a teaching tool in addition to being a tool for the purposes of evaluation. If this is not done, much of the educational value of the test is completely lost.

## SUMMARY

In this chapter we have tried to help the reader grasp the importance of evaluation in nursing education, to acquaint her with a frame of reference for constructing and utilizing tests effectively, and to discuss some procedures found useful in the construction of classroom tests. We have emphasized that two questions provide us with a handy frame of reference for constructing tests: What decisions do I want the test results to help me to make? What data do I need in order to make these decisions?

We have also looked at some of the different kinds of tests which may be used to call forth and provide us with a record of the behavioral samples which will be used in making decisions. We have looked at the following items: single answer, completion, multiple choice, true-false, matching, classification, identification, listing, essay, oral, and situation or problem solving. For each of these items we have examined the differentiating characteristics, the advantages and limitations associated with their use, and the guidelines which facilitate the construction of such items. In addition, we have considered some factors associated with the assembling of the test, the utilization of instructions, the use of answer sheets, and the use of a test as a teaching tool.

To paraphrase a statement by Thorndike and Hagen, we may know the quality of an instructor by the tests she creates and administers. They tell what she is truly valuing in her students, even though she herself does not know it, and they influence profoundly what her students will learn.

# Chapter 10

# Clinical Evaluation

The process of evaluation in the clinical area is perhaps the most difficult task faced by most nursing educators. Part of this difficulty lies in the fact that clinical evaluation seems to be highly ambiguous in nature, and to be particularly vulnerable to problems of subjectivity and instructor bias. By clinical evaluation we refer to the process of assessing student progress in all educational experiences outside of formal classroom or didactic situations. It particularly refers to a student's ability to provide safe, competent nursing care under supervision to patients. Another difficulty results from the proposition that clinical evaluation is perhaps the most important dimension in the assessment of student learning, since at no other time will the student likely be as closely supervised and a detailed evaluation made of her competence in the clinical area. A review of the literature in nursing education indicates that grades in the clinical area, objectives of clinical evaluation, techniques for assessing student progress, are among the most widely discussed concerns in nursing education today among students, nursing educators, and nurse practitioners.

Several problem areas seem to highlight the current situation. The first of these revolves around discrepancies between faculty expectations of students and the expectations of nurse practitioners. The second deals with the discrepancy between students' objectives and those of the nursing faculty. For example, in the first area, Bohan (1967) found no significant relation between the grades of baccalaureate nursing students in nursing courses, and the students' performance as professional nurses as measured through self- and supervisory evaluations. Smith (1965) and Redman (1964) both found conflicting expectations and emphases between nursing faculty and nursing service. The resulting conflicts frequently leave the student caught in the middle. On the one hand, she is evaluated by what she feels are the idealistic standards of the faculty. On the other, she constantly views around her in the clinical area the wide divergence in techniques, practices, and attitudes used or expressed by staff nurses and supervisory personnel. The resulting contradictions in the student's mind seem to be one of the main contributing forces to the disillusionment students frequently feel at some stage of their program.

This same conflict was evidenced in differing student-faculty attitudes and expectations. For example, Redman (1968) found that students felt that their relations with their patients were clearly more important than those with clinical instructors or other students. Seivwright (1968) added to this the finding that student expectations concerning

*141*

their clinical experiences differed substantially from those held by their instructors. She also found a sizable number of nursing students who held negative or uncertain attitudes about the worth and objectives of their clinical experience. In both studies the importance of a thorough orientation of nursing staff and students prior to the commencement of any clinical experience seems to be clearly indicated. Such an orientation would include educational objectives, planned experiences, time sequences, and methods of evaluation. If we hope to make the clinical experience a valued and integral part of the learning process, then there needs to be initial agreement on the objectives to be reached, and the roles of faculty, students, and nursing staff as contributors to reaching these objectives.

## THE QUALIFICATION PROCESS

Before one can begin to evaluate, it is necessary to determine clearly the goals to be reached and the methods to be used in assisting students to reach these goals. In addition, we need to include the specific objectives the student needs to meet in satisfying the goals, and the behavior she is expected to demonstrate. Evaluation does not occur until later, when we wish to assess the student's ability to perform in the desired way and for the desired reasons. Therefore it seems logical in our discussion of clinical evaluation in this chapter to proceed in an orderly fashion from the initial setting of goals to the final evaluation conferences between faculty and students. This process is designed to enable both the students and faculty to learn and grow together in a mutually helpful relationship, i.e. the faculty members sharing with the students their skills, knowledge, understandings, objectives, and so forth, and the students sharing with the faculty their concerns, their reactions to the learning process, and their self-assessment of their progress and problems.

The procedure we have been pointing toward may be best understood under the title of a qualification process, i.e. a process designed to assist each student to qualify as a safe, competent graduate nurse. Perhaps the best way of understanding this process is to apply it to an actual situation. The faculty members in an associate degree nursing program were unhappy about their current clinical evaluation procedures and decided to revise the entire system. The first step in a qualification system involves the entire faculty in the setting of program objectives. These objectives must be specific, and represent the best thinking of the faculty. Before they are adopted, the entire faculty must make any revisions necessary so that the final product is agreed to by all.

After this procedure the 11 faculty members in the AD program met to develop better procedures for clinical assessment. Prior to this meeting the faculty were following a previously developed statement of philosophy. This included a list of 11 program objectives to be achieved by the graduates of the school, each of which was followed by a list of desired behaviors that varied from specific objectives to idealized attitudes that were almost impossible to assess. Working together as a to-tal group, the faculty finally agreed on two new broad objectives to be met by each graduate from the school. These new objectives en-compassed the best elements of the original 11.

In the second stage of a qualification system, broad objectives are then subdivided into a series of highly specific behavioral objectives, following the model previously described in Chapter 8. These behavioral objectives should then represent the guidelines for the program. This step was followed by the faculty in the AD program. The faculty members separated into work groups according to their teaching as-signment—first year and second year. Each group of faculty members took the new broad objectives and utilized them in analyzing each course in the particular year. Thus the first-year faculty members translated the broad objectives into specific objectives for each course. These objectives were written in the form of behavioral criteria designed to lead sequentially from initial entrance in the program to graduation. Any item that in the judgment of the faculty could not be assessed objectively was eliminated. The remaining items for all practical purposes became a curriculum guide for the faculty to follow in planning appropriate clinical experiences. In addition, there was an important component prior to actual evaluation that needs to be discussed at this time.

## MINIMAL COMPETENCY AND DESIRABLE PERFORMANCE

We recognize that in any body of knowledge there are some things one must know, and other things that would be desirable to know. The "must know" or minimal competency includes that specific knowledge or safe level of performance that the student must demonstrate if she is to be permitted to progress or graduate. To put it another way, this mini-mal competency represents the pass level—if the student does not know it or cannot demonstrate it, she fails. Our hope as educators would be twofold: to help each student go as far as possible beyond the level of minimal competency, and to try to prevent persistent minimal com-petency by able students. Through a qualification process both faculty and students are committed to the same goal—to help each student successfully complete her program. If the student meets the level of minimal competency, she qualifies; if she does not, she does not qualify. This is assuming that she has been allowed ample opportunity for re-petitions of the experience to obtain the minimal standard.

In the AD program mentioned earlier, the faculty completed the first stages by subdividing the broad objectives into specific course objec-tives, and then defining these course objectives in concrete behavioral terms, each of which could be assessed. At the same time the faculty assigned to work at each level went through the behavioral objectives and skills, and designated those that all agreed were necessary for mini-mal competency. To cite one illustration, the ability to measure the pro-per dose of a medication was considered part of minimal competency. The knowledge of the history of the profession of nursing was con-sidered desirable, but not mandatory. Thus, if the student failed the history material, she was still allowed to progress in the program. The items and areas that comprised the level of minimal competency formed the core of the curriculum and planned clinical experience within each course. In addition, they were carefully explained to students at the beginning of each course, along with the criteria and methods to be used in determining whether in fact a student had achieved at least minimal competency. For those schools utilizing a pass-fail or satisfactory-unsatisfactory grading system in the clinical area, this level of minimal competency represents the cut-off point below which a student fails.

There are several points to keep in mind in setting up such a qualification system. First, this system is not meant to suggest that we should be content with allowing students merely to demonstrate minimal competencies. By working cooperatively with each student toward the qualification goal, we concentrate in helping her grow and learn to her full capacity. We are more interested in each student's personal growth toward qualification than we are in comparing her with her classmates. Second, we have found that the qualification system based on minimal competency sharply reduces the assessment problems of the faculty and the threat of evaluation for the students. It tends to reduce significantly the academic games usually played between faculty and students, for both now clearly know the mandatory material required to demonstrate minimal competency, and the criteria that will be used for assessment. Instead, both faculty and students are now working together toward common goals.

Third, an essential part of the qualification process rests on an effective feedback or progress report system. This places the responsibility upon each faculty member to share constantly with each student her progress toward meeting the stated objectives of each course or clinical experience. Without going into great detail at this point, if a student reaches the end of a course or clinical experience, and is surprised by her failure, the faculty may have failed completely to provide the proper kind of ongoing criticism so that the student is aware at all times of her progress. Since there is no standard mandatory or minimal competency in nursing education, competency must be determined and agreed to by all the faculty members in an area within a particular program.

Assuming that faculty members have worked through the stages described above, we are now ready to move to the next step, i.e. beginning to create an environment in which students are able to demonstrate their growing ability and clinical skills. In most cases the student's academic knowledge has been assessed previously in the classroom setting through paper-and-pencil tests. Now the problem becomes one of providing opportunities for the student to demonstrate that she has the ability to apply correctly the knowledge she has learned in class.

## FEEDBACK AND THE QUALIFICATION PROCESS

To make a qualification process work, faculty members should be able to help each other and the students, and students should be able to help each other and the faculty to reach the desired goals in the most efficient way possible. Both faculty members and students need to know what they are doing well, where they can improve, and, whenever possible, ways in which they can improve or change their behavior. We should, however, recognize that frequently there are barriers to giving and receiving assistance from someone else.

1. It is difficult to admit our deficiencies even to ourselves. It may be even harder to admit them to someone else. There are concerns sometimes whether we can really trust the other person, particularly if it is a clinical or other professional situation which might have an effect on our standing. We may also be afraid of what the other person thinks of us.

2. We may have struggled so hard to make ourselves independent persons that the thought of depending on another person seems to violate something within us. Or we may all of our lives have looked for someone on whom to be dependent, and we try to repeat this pattern in our relation with those around us.

3. We may be looking for sympathy and support rather than for help in seeing our difficulty more clearly. We ourselves may have to change, as well as others in the situation. When the other person tries to point out some of the ways we are contributing to the problem, we may stop listening. Solving a problem may mean uncovering some of the sides of ourselves which we have avoided or wished to avoid thinking about.

4. We may feel that our problem or situation is so unique that no one could ever understand it, and certainly not an outsider.

Barriers to giving assistance are as follows:

1. Most of us like to give advice. Doing so suggests to us that we are competent and important. We easily get caught in a telling role without testing whether our advice is appropriate to the abilities, the fears or the power of the person we are trying to help.

2. If the person we are trying to help becomes defensive, we may try to argue with or pressure her, i.e. meet resistance with more pressure which increases resistance. This is typical in arguments.

3. We may confuse the relationship by responding to only one aspect of what we see in the other person's problem by overpraising, avoiding the recognition that the person being helped must see not only her strengths, but also the areas she needs to change or improve.

The foregoing points apply to both students and faculty members, each of whom may assume either role with the other, or among themselves. There are certain qualities which serve to minimize or eliminate the artificial barriers that are thrown up between people. These are as follows:

1. Mutual trust

2. Recognition that the helping situation is a joint responsibility

3. Listening, with the helper listening more than the person receiving help

4. Behavior by the helper which is calculated to make it easier for the person receiving help to talk.

At the heart of the qualification system is the process of feedback mentioned earlier. Interpersonal feedback is a way of helping another person to consider changing her behavior. It is communication to a person or a group which gives that person information about how she is performing or how she affects others. The feed-back process must involve all the members within a school of nursing to be effective. This includes faculty feedback to each other, student feedback to each other, and faculty-student feedback to each other. Ideally it is a two-way communication; i.e. the receiver needs to know how she is perceived by the sender; the sender needs to know how she can more effectively communicate with or help the receiver. The more open and honest we can each be with those around us, the easier it becomes for everyone to give more effective feedback. Some useful criteria for feedback are as follows:

1. It is descriptive rather than evaluative. By describing one's own reaction, it leaves the person free to use it or not to use it as she sees fit. By avoiding evaluative language, e.g. using adverbs instead of adjectives, it reduces the need for the person to react defensively.

2. It is specific rather than general. To be told that one is "dominating" will probably not be as useful as to be told, "Just now when we were discussing the problem in the group, I felt that you did not listen to what others said, and I felt forced to accept your arguments or face attack from you."

3. It includes the needs of both the receiver and the giver of feedback. Feedback can be destructive when it serves only our own needs and fails to consider the needs of the person on the receiving end.

4. It is directed toward behavior which the receiver can do something about. Frustration is only increased when a person is reminded of some shortcoming over which she has no control.

5. Feedback is most useful when the receiver has evaluated herself, and then has formulated the kind of question which those observing her can answer; i.e. asking for feedback from others may be a way of also giving feedback, e.g., "I get the feeling that you are not interested in what I am saying—is there something I can do that might help you more?"

If feedback is not asked for, it still should be given to ensure that a person has the knowledge of a deficiency and the opportunity to change. It may be desirable to ask first whether the person would like to receive feedback, e.g., "I have noticed some specific things which seem to be interfering with your performance. I'd like to share them with you because you may find them useful," or, "I notice that you haven't asked for feedback for a while from me—I wonder if there is something I do which makes it difficult for you to ask."

6. In general, feedback is most useful at the earliest opportunity after the given behavior (depending, of course, on the person's readiness to hear it, support available from others, and so forth).

7. One way to check clear communication is to have the receiver try to rephrase the feedback she has received to see whether it corresponds to what the sender had in mind. For example, ask the receiver to think about what has been said, and briefly write out her understanding of it.

8. When feedback is given to a member of a group, both the giver and the receiver have the opportunity to check with others in the group

the accuracy of the feedback. Is this just one person's impression, or is the impression shared with others?

## SIMULATED LEARNING

One common problem that occurs in all the helping professions re- volves around the point at which students are ready to begin work with people, i.e. patients, clients, counselors, and others. We have a re- sponsibility to the person for whom we are providing help or care to en- sure that he is not harmed by the assistance given by a student who is learning. Because of this, faculty members in the helping professions have been placing increasing emphasis upon intermediary steps between the classroom and the bedside. These steps seem to fall into two broad interrelated areas. The first involves the development of some sort of simulated clinical or laboratory experience. The second involves the use of practice techniques such as role playing. Neither method is perfect, but both seem to provide natural transitions for students moving into the clinical area. They also allow the faculty to maintain the de- velopmental process of the student gradually moving toward minimal competency in the desired areas.

*Role playing* has been widely used in the helping professions, particularly those that rely heavily on verbal and nonverbal com- munication between individuals and groups. This may be done in several ways, depending on the skill to be practiced. Perhaps the best method is to develop sequential role playing. As a first step, a demonstration of the techniques to be practiced may be held in front of a group. Typically, at least one faculty member is involved as one of the participants in the role-playing situation. If those doing the dem- onstration are all students, they must practice in advance so that the proper techniques are shown to the group. In general, the most effective initial demonstration utilizes the faculty member as the nurse, counselor, therapist, or the like.

After the initial demonstration the group of students may be broken into subgroups of three. The primary advantage of triads lies in the fact that one student can play the role of the nurse, one the patient, and one can observe. After the role playing session the three can discuss what happened and why. Then the students can switch roles until each has had an opportunity to function in each role. After the subgroups have practiced, the entire class can then come back together to discuss prob- lems, feelings, and what they feel they have learned.

Simulated learning experiences are not unusual in nursing education. Simplified versions of these may be found in the case studies and problem-solving situations given to students in classroom tests and exercises. These problem-solving exercises are beginning to expand more into the clinical area. Several examples reported in the nursing education literature serve to illustrate this point.

Bitzer (1966) reports on the development of a computer-controlled teaching system for use in nursing education. A portion of a medical- surgical nursing study unit was programmed for use on the computer system. It was presented to six students who obtained information by themselves in the PLATO simulated laboratory, while seven students served as a control in regular classes with a regular instructor. A comparison of post-test results on subject-matter knowledge showed a significant difference at the 0.09 level in favor of the PLATO group. The use of a computer system to provide a simulated laboratory allowed students to proceed at their own pace. Student response to this sort of learning was very favorable.

Simpson (1967) describes the current use of the "walk-around" laboratory practical examination. A series of nursing stations are set up to test out a series of judgments. Students are provided with an answer sheet on which to write their responses as they move from one station to another answering questions written on a card attached to a clinical implement or entity. The time allowed at each station is limited and clocked by an instructor. This same technique can be used in a variety of ways.

Tornyay (1968) describes the Simulated Clinical Nursing Problem Test. The problem is introduced with a description of the patient, the medical diagnosis, and physician's orders. The students are told that they will care for the mock patient for several days. Students find this test lifelike, and are upset when they learn that they have made faulty decisions about the patient's care. The test is designed to measure problem-solving ability. Since there is little, if any, room for error when working with actual patients, this test allows the student to exercise her judgment, and be informed of the consequences of her actions without direct patient contact or risk.

Frejlach and Corcoran (1971) seem to sum up this phase of our discussion by their report of a method developed to evaluate a student's clinical performance. Slides, movies, audiotapes and videotapes, role playing, and simulated clinical situations are all used to test the students' abilities. Some parts are administered individually; others to small groups. Each item was pretested and had established criteria. Overall, this seems to combine many of the better elements previously described. These simulated experiences are designed to help students develop clinical judgment. While experiencing these, students are also gradually being exposed to actual patient care, at the same time utilizing simple techniques such as TPR, and others.

## SELECTION OF LEARNING ACTIVITIES

As we move into the area of planning for a variety of learning experiences, the question occurs in the clinical area as to the best method of planning appropriate activities for students. The faculty has already developed clear-cut objectives and expressed these in behavioral terms. These have been clearly communicated to the students so that both faculty and students know the objectives and the logical steps to be followed in achieving these objectives. In order to plan the appropriate learning activities in the clinical setting, the instructor is now faced with several problems. One is the lack of a sufficient number of appropriate patients with whom students may work, and the other is how best to select patients with whom students may work.

Galeener (1966) described the problems encountered in providing meaningful clinical experiences. These were the availability of patients on any one clinical setting having problems directly related to classroom content, and the gradual increase in the number of students that each instructor must work with at any one time in each clinical experience. She describes a group method by which two to four students are assigned to the care of a single patient, and thus fewer appropriate patients are needed to provide meaningful learning experience. The trap in this approach lies in the potential for segmented learning on the part of students, i.e. where each student is assigned to a certain kind of care. This problem can be overcome, however, by stressing the concept of team nursing, and also by having each student on the team care for the total patient, while the others observe.

We are still left with the second problem, that of selecting patients to be cared for by students. Patient selection becomes vitally important if students are to gain the proper experiences under our previously described qualification system. Normally, the instructor has selected the patients in each clinical sequence, but this unilateral decision has been challenged by at least three different authors. Kramer (1967) attempted to examine differences between clinical experiences selected by students and those selected by an instructor. She found that students tended to select experiences comparable to those selected by instructors. An important area of differentiation was that students tended to select patients whom they perceived as having communication stress or anxiety, while instructor selections involved a wider range of problems, including physiological and psychological. She feels that greater student involvement is needed in the planning and selection of learning activities if the student is to be helped to develop a greater feeling of responsibility toward learning.

McCaffery (1968) suggests that students should choose their own patients. Objectives and performance goals are given to students in advance, so that the student knows what she is to learn in the clinical area, and she can assume some degree of responsibility for her own learning. Treece (1969) found similar results in a study which indicated that two thirds of the student sample indicated a desire to assume at least some responsibility for patient selection, although students seemed unwilling to assume full responsibility for selection as they gained clinical experience. In general, if the learning process is truly a team effort between the instructor and the student, then both should be involved in selecting and planning the appropriate learning experiences in the clinical area.

## METHODS OF SUPERVISION

It is not the purpose of this book to concentrate on curriculum planning or techniques of supervision. It is important, however, to mention several points at this time because they have a direct bearing upon the effectiveness of learning and the assessment of progress in the clinical area. We recognize that the more threatening the evaluation and supervision process becomes, the less students are able to learn and perform. For example, students frequently wonder whether or not they ever do anything right, for the only time they ever hear from an instructor is when they have made a mistake. Komorita (1965) found a common pattern in which students reported that they liked the security of having the instructor readily available, but felt they were being observed and supervised to excess. Essentially, they complain that someone is always watching them and "breathing down their necks." Cautela (1964) reports on a different dynamic in which some students are threatened by their supervisors or instructors to the point at which they begin to feel that the worst will happen to them. This self-fulfilling prophecy creates many fears and anxieties which hinder individual clinical performance. A great deal of student counseling is done precisely over this matter.

Zasowska (1967) dealt with other problems in her research study. She found that clinical laboratory experiences do not always complement course or class content; the focus of the clinical experience too often rests on a specific nursing activity, losing sight of the educational objective; the patient rather than the individual student seems to be the main focus of attention; the student's readiness to begin a clinical experience is usually assumed; and the evaluation of learning is not an integral part of each clinical experience.

Perhaps the most common method of clinical supervision used at present is that provided by an instructor who is there watching a student perform certain tasks. This has the advantage of having the instructor readily available to assist the student if she gets into difficulty, and enables the instructor to be aware of everything the student does. It has the disadvantage of changing the dynamics of the situation. The student is well aware of the presence of her instructor, and may not react as she would normally. The patient will frequently try to support or protect the student if the instructor is present. This approach may be the safest one for supervision, but it is of debatable effectiveness in observing communication skills or student-patient interaction. It also limits the amount of experience a student may have because the instructor can observe only one or two students closely at any given time.

The foregoing method also introduces some of the problems mentioned previously relating to supervision. For example, some faculty members observe students in the clinical area to help integrate the physical and emotional aspects of patient care. Yet much of their time initially must be spent trying to work through students' feelings about supervision, and the tendency to view the integrator with suspicion. In an effort to avoid some of these problems, instructors may rely heavily on clinical conferences, during which the group has the opportunity to talk through their experiences of the day and, most importantly, their feelings about the experiences. These are an excellent way for students to learn from each other in a free and open environment, provided the post conferences do not become evaluation tools. The students' ability to recall their daily experiences and interventions during the post conferences will depend on the removal of threat on the part of the instructor.

This leads us to the second method, which at least supplements the foregoing method of supervision, and in some instances may be the primary method used. We refer here to student self-reports of what occurred during the clinical experience or a particular nursing intervention. These may take several forms and operate under several names. Hamm and Hartsfield (1970) report on a variation of the self-report in a description of students' reactions to the clinical experience. Each week, students were asked to submit information about their personal appraisals of (1) teacher behavior which increased motivation, (2) teacher behavior which decreased motivation, (3) classmate behavior which increased motivation, and (4) classmate behavior which decreased motivation. It is of interest to note that students tended to be more specific in identifying teacher behaviors that decreased motivation. Also, students who interpreted the hostility of an instructor as unjustifiable tended to retaliate by refraining from study or discussion.

The more normal sort of self-report deals with student reports of their nursing care in clinical situations. One example of these is *process recording*. Nehren and Batey (1963) define process recording as "the verbatim and seriatim recording to the extent that memory will permit of the verbal and non-verbal interaction that has occurred between the patient and the nurse." This method is useful in removing the physical threat of the instructor, but students are seldom able to remember everything that occurred. Many important facets of the interaction may be lost. Students also get defensive and tend to cover up or gloss over areas in which they know they did poorly.

Nevertheless, despite its defects, process recording can still be an invaluable teaching tool. Good process recordings contain the student's feelings and analysis of patient care and interaction. The student expression of her feelings serves as an excellent focal point for counseling in the clinical area as the student talks about what she has written, reconstructs what happened, and begins to share her feelings about the interaction and herself. Students tend to object to the work involved in these process recordings or other self-reports, but they later appreciate them as a growth experience when used within reason.

Tadlock (1964) describes the requirement that students write an *interaction study*. The study necessitated the active participation of the student in the clinical situation, rather than the mere reporting of facts, which is the usual situation in reporting only anecdotal material. The study enabled the student to share her feelings about each situation and to clarify the motives for her behavior. Although called by a different name, the procedure essentially is a variation of process recording.

Crowley (1965) discusses the use of the *clinical diary* to provide the instructor with continuous first-hand data upon which to base class discussions, and to provide the student with a running record of thoughts or events in the clinical area. The diaries helped to integrate classroom and clinical material. They proved to be beneficial in correcting problems that arose during the clinical experience, and gave valuable evidence as to how much and in what way the students were using class concepts in patient care. Again, this seems to combine many of the elements of process recording and post-clinical conferences.

Another method of self-report deals with the student writing of *anecdotal records*. Several authors report the use of such records as a method of self-evaluation. Palmer (1963) relates that students in one school are required to write at least one anecdote a week during their medical-surgical course. The anecdote should include reactions to nursing measures, evaluation of performance, thoughts on the nurse-patient interview, interpersonal or communication problems, and statements of personal feelings. Some instructors decided not to write anecdotal records of their own, but to add to the students'. The anecdotes provided instructors with insights and information otherwise unavailable. Self-assessment also helped many students to arrive at the conclusion that they were unsuited for nursing. A similar process is described by Palmer (1967). The more common practice of instructors preparing anecdotal material will be discussed a little later.

Lenz and Bauer (1970) combine several of the foregoing descriptions in what is called a *nursing care study*. In other places this is sometimes called a *nursing care plan*. These utilize many of the techniques described above. Every student maintains a comprehensive study on each patient under her care. This study includes the detailed plan for patient care, process recordings, and clinical diary entries. Here again, the main emphasis was placed on self-reporting and self-analysis of the student's ability to plan and carry out competent, safe nursing care.

Schultz (1964) describes a variation of self-report. In her situation, instructors write anecdotal reports, including any observations that seem pertinent to patient care. These are available to students throughout the quarter. In addition, students keep a clinical diary of their first three days' experience in psychiatric nursing. Students are also expected to use a self-evaluation tool, using a scale of 1 to 7 related to clinical objectives with supporting examples. Although Schultz feels that anecdotal records are time-consuming, rely too much on memory, and are too subjective, they do serve a purpose when combined with self-evaluation measures and counseling.

## AUDIOVISUAL AIDS

Both methods described above—physical supervision and self-reporting—represent the most common kinds of clinical supervision in use today. There is beginning to be a rapid increase, however, in the use of audiovisual techniques as a supervisory and evaluative tool. Nursing educators have long relied on the use of films, slides, and similar techniques in classroom teaching. With the advent of portable videotape units, more is being done in utilizing videotape recordings as teaching tools. This practice is not particularly new. One example was reported by Westley and Hornback in 1964. They felt that basic skills in nursing could be taught by means of videotapes. They found advantages to both students and faculty in the use of such equipment. The advantages to the student included consistently organized and easily viewed lessons which could be reinforced and supplemented by the instructor. The instructor in turn does not have to spend her time collecting and testing equipment before a demonstration; she knows the exact time necessary to view the demonstration; and she has additional time for other teaching activities.

Videotaping has not yet been widely used in the clinical area. The method is almost standard practice in many other helping professions, such as the training of counselors, social workers, teachers, and others. There are several possible examples of potential use in nursing education. A portable camera and videotape recorder could be used in home visits or in selected clinical situations, always with the permission of the patient. Those schools of nursing that have access to a clinical unit which monitors individual patients by closed-circuit television can hook a videotape recorder into the master control unit. Although initially costly in terms of equipment ($1500 to $2000 per unit would be the current range), this method has the greatest promise for clinical teaching and supervision. An instructor who is able to view the videotape of a student caring for a patient with that student is able to point out verbal and nonverbal behavior more effectively than ever before. The student can also view the tape herself or with classmates as an additional reinforcement to learning.

For those schools without the facilities or the funds to utilize videotape techniques, there is one alternative available for clinical supervision that has been used for some time, particularly in psychiatric nursing—this is the use of audiotapes. Smith (1970) and Stevens (1970) both report similar uses of audiotapes. Students taped home interviews in the clinical experience in community nursing. Smith found it useful not to tape the first two interviews. The patients gave their written permission for taping on forms provided. Students evaluated their performance on the taped interview, and added information about nonverbal communication. Instructors listened to the tapes, reviewed the students' self-evaluation, and added their comments about how well the student seemed to use sound principles of interviewing and teaching. After review the instructor went over the tape with the student. With the student's permission, tapes were also used for small group discussion. This same method can be used effectively in any kind of patient care that relies heavily on verbal interaction. It will not be too useful in clinical evaluation of actual nursing care except in psychiatry and public health nursing, nor is it ideal in portraying nonverbal communication. Playing back the tapes also takes a great deal of time. Nevertheless it is perhaps the best substitute we currently have for videotaping in providing an accurate picture of an actual student-patient interaction.

## INSTRUCTOR REPORTS

Up to this point we have been primarily discussing self-report techniques as well as methods of gathering information about student progress and learning. Just as learning is a two-way process between faculty and students, so is the gathering of evaluative information. Faculty members are charged with the responsibility of ultimately determining a student's ability to function in a competent, safe manner in the clinical area. In order to do this, they need all the information possible. This information may be gathered and reported in several ways. One way includes anecdotal material based on systematic observation, as well as structured interviews. The other includes more structured written methods, including rating scales and behavioral check lists.

*Anecdotal records* are one of the most frequently used data-collecting devices for observation and evaluation of student behavior. A good anecdote is brief and specific, and contains the following elements:

1. It provides an actual description of an actual event.

2. It describes the setting where the event or incident occurred sufficiently to give the incident meaning.

3. Interpretation or the instructor's opinion is separated from the factual description and clearly identified.

4. The event or incident described is usually one that relates to the student's personal and professional development or social interaction.

5. The event reported is either representative of the typical behavior of the student, or is significant because it is strikingly atypical for the student.

The anecdotal record can best be used in reporting conversation and interpersonal relationships, in which variations in situations and personalities preclude any advance determination of behavior. Anecdotal material can also be used to record specific short incidents illustrating a student's use of nursing skills and techniques or of judgment, in order to show trends in her behavior. Keeping the instructor's opinion separate from the anecdote frees anyone else reading the incident to form her own opinion based on the facts presented.

The anecdotal record lends itself well to frequent observations of short duration. One anecdote by itself is of little or no value, but a series of notes can be helpful in pointing up persistent trends or behaviors over a period of time. Too often the instructor is tempted to record a mixture of fact and opinion rather than keeping them separate. Ideally, there should be a number of anecdotes written by different instructors about each student over a period of time. By using more than one source of anecdotes, individual bias tends to be minimized. Maintaining good anecdotal records can also be a large clerical burden for an already overloaded faculty. This problem can be greatly lessened by providing dictating equipment so that instructors can dictate anecdotal material to be transcribed later by a secretary.

It is important that anecdotal records be made available for students to review at any time. They should be periodically summarized and individual reports destroyed. It takes practice to write good anecdotes. A good in-service training program for a faculty is to write some anecdotes, share them with other faculty members, and ask for specific criticism. Each instructor should be particularly looking at the way the anecdote is interpreted by each reader. If there are sharp differences in meaning, then the anecdotal record is probably too ambiguous or subjective. As mentioned earlier, anecdotal material is widely used in nursing education. As an addendum to the point already made of giving students ready on-going access to anecdotes written about them, it is important to remember that students need the opportunity to discuss anecdotes with instructors at regular intervals. Berzon (1970) reports an example of a final evaluation written almost entirely from anecdotal material.

Besides formal or structured instruments, there was only one other method reported in the literature to obtain information about a student's performance in the clinical setting. Murphy (1971) reports on the use of a structured interview in a community health course. Students were evaluated in two ways. Each family was interviewed by an instructor for its assessment of the students' activities, and students' records of what they had done with their families were examined. This adds a potentially valuable new dimension to student evaluation. The involvement of patients and their families in the educational process has much merit, and should be explored further by nursing educators.

Marilyn L. Dyer suggested the possibility of patient evaluation in her talk at the 1970 Regional Workshops of the Council of Diploma Programs of NLN. She stated:

> There are some mechanical problems in obtaining evaluations of the students from (patients); however, effort should be made to devise some type of questionnaire that would elicit such information as to how the patient was made comfortable, whether the student gave the patient a feeling of being secure and having his needs met, etc. Here is the individual who should really be consulted for evaluation purposes—"the consumer of nursing care." Yet, how many times is such an excellent source of data overlooked.

Dyer adds one other interesting point—that head nurses and supervisors may also be asked to participate in the evaluation of a student, using many of the tools described in this chapter. Dyer's suggestions are well worth considering for additional aids to evaluation.


## RATING SCALES

Perhaps the most common method currently in use in clinical evaluation to arrive at a grade is the *rating scale*. A rating scale has two main features: (1) a description of the characteristics to be rated, and (2) some means by which the instructor may indicate the quality, frequency or importance of each item. A good rating scale has the following characteristics:

1. It is important to determine specifically what you are trying to find out. As previously discussed, the initial setting of clinical objectives is a critical first step in any educational planning. We need to know curricular emphases, and also, as previously described, which emphases represent minimal competencies. As Palmer (1962) pointed out, well defined, mutually shared clinical objectives lead to much greater consistency in evaluation.

2. Faculty members must then determine, based on the clinical objectives, the most effective ways of measuring those things that can be measured. We must recognize that certain attitudes and characteristics are difficult, if not impossible, to measure, despite the fact that they are important. For example, we may feel that commitment to nursing as a profession may be an important consideration in assessing the overall performance of a student. Nevertheless, at our present level of sophistication in measurement, we have no valid way to measure this. We may also have to recognize that some things may be better measured through classroom tests, while others can be effectively assessed only through clinical observation.

3. The scale contains clearly defined traits, expressed in the form of brief descriptions of behavior that can be observed. This takes us back to our previous discussion of specific behavioral objectives. These can be related directly to a rating scale. Our only reasonable clues as to what a student is are in terms of her behavior. Evaluating behavior tends to be unreliable because behaviors under observation tend to be complex and variable. Both the faculty member and the student are constantly changing, and the behavioral criteria used on scales are at best samples of behavior at the moment. The more specific is the behavioral objective on the scale, the more easily and validly is it assessed.

4. Space should be provided on the scale for the faculty member to record instances or anecdotes that will support the rating given. This procedure tends to minimize the arbitrary nature of some ratings.

5. The faculty member should be encouraged to indicate on the form when she has had no opportunity to observe the specific behavioral item to be rated. When space is not provided, faculty members tend to rate in the average range rather than leave the item blank.

6. The scale should be limited to behavioral items chosen because of their importance. Too often, scales include a wide mixture of items ranging from very important to comparitively unimportant. If the scale assesses behaviors in several areas, the areas should be weighted in terms of their relative importance to each other.

7. The scale should be accompanied with specific directions for completing the form. This will help in reducing the ambiguity of terms and behavioral criteria.

8. Both the scale and the instructions for completion should be developed in cooperation with those who will use the form. This is vitally important. Just as the specific behavioral objectives should be developed by all the faculty responsible for meeting those objectives, so should any tool for evaluation be developed by all those who will use the tool.

9. Whenever possible, utilize four categories on the rating scale rather than five in order to force faculty members to discriminate by placing students in other than a middle or average category. For example, categories in groups of four, such as superior, above average, average, low; or always, usually, sometimes, seldom; or high, above average, below average, low, are much easier to rate and to obtain inter-rater consistency than groups of five categories. As a general rule, the fewer the categories, the more reliable are the ratings.

The building of a good rating scale takes time and effort on the part of a faculty. A series of brief scales is more desirable to measure specific skills, while broader categories can be used to measure behavior common to all clinical situations, such as nurse-patient relations. A good deal has been written describing the steps in the construction of good rating scales. For example, Hazeltine and Zetz (1964) describe a five-point scale which used 0 for unsafe practice, 1 for safe with intensive guidance, 2 met the objective of the clinical experience with moderate guidance, 3 met the objective of the clinical experience with minimum guidance, and 4 met the objective of the clinical experience with unusual self-direction.

Ortelt (1966) describes a scale that provides ample space for supportive statements of an anecdotal nature which would greatly increase the value of the rating. O'Shea (1967) gives one of the better descriptions of the construction of a scale. The faculty members of an AD program developed the philosophy and objectives of the nursing program, and translated these into behavioral changes that were expected to occur. Four broad areas were selected for rating: the student performs in a safe manner, the student understands the reasons underlying patient care, the student develops patient-centered relationships, and the student possesses the personal and intellectual qualities important to nursing. Criteria were developed for the evaluation of each of these areas.

Shield (1968) describes scales that either run from 1 to 10 or are open and continuous. The University of Arizona (1970) presented a detailed plan for developing a rating instrument which included plans for revising the scale. This should be done regularly because of the constant turnover in nursing faculty, to ensure that the objectives and the scale still represent the thinking of the current group of faculty members. Moritz and Sexton (1970) describe a scale that assesses behavior in five broad areas: planning, implementing, interpersonal relationships, communication, and evaluation. They also describe a weighting procedure for each area. Durham (1970) describes the process of developing 96 statements contributed by nursing faculty expressed in behavioral terms, and grouped into five distinct areas. Dunn (1970) also describes the construction and validation of a rating instrument, but comments on the problem of the lack of relation between ratings and classroom tests.

Although much has been written about the development of rating scales, it is entirely possible that such scales may be completely unnecessary for clinical evaluation. In Chapter 8 we discussed the advantages of a satisfactory-unsatisfactory or pass-fail system in the clinical area. This is being reported more and more frequently in the nursing literature. Earlier in this chapter we also discussed a qualification system based on minimal competencies and desirable knowledge. If a school of nursing is using this sort of system, there is no need for the use of rating scales. Instead, a simple check list of behaviors and skills broken into minimal competency and desired behaviors will serve the purpose of evaluation without the problems inherent in building, validating, and using rating scales.

## CHECK LISTS AND OTHER TOOLS

Brester et al. (1962) described the process in developing an *evaluation guide* for a medical-surgical course. The end-product was a somewhat open-ended form divided into three columns. The first column identified the general objectives for the course. The second listed the specific learning areas for each objective. The third provided the identifiable behavioral criteria for meeting each objective. The final form resembles a semistructured anecdotal record system based on behavioral criteria.

Anderson (1968) describes one example of the use of a *check list.* The particular form presented dealt with a tool to evaluate moving and positioning patients from supine to side-lying positions based on the Hoffman method. The check list consists of two parts. The observation sheet is the actual check list for recording the observable behaviors in the activity. The criteria sheet identifies the specific criteria to be used in evaluating the student's success or failure on each item on the check list. Although it might be desirable to have one evaluative instrument that could cover the gamut of nursing activities, it may be necessary to develop a series of check lists to evaluate smaller segments of behavior.

As mentioned earlier, the success or failure of a good check list tends to rest on the grading system used in the clinical area. If the faculty in a school can reach consensus on clinical objectives, behavioral criteria, a grading system based on pass-fail or satisfactory-unsatisfactory, and behavior that represents minimal competency, then one or more check lists may solve our problems of evaluation in the clinical area. On each item on the list the instructor just checks off when a student has demonstrated at least minimal mastery of a particular skill or technique. In order to pass, the student must complete satisfactorily all mandatory items in the clinical sequence. Ideally, the student would be checked on each item or skill in different situations by different clinical instructors, but this may not always be possible. Nevertheless a good safeguard can be built in by requesting that another instructor observe a potentially failing student as a validity check.

Check lists have been found to work effectively in highly specialized clinical areas. With faculty involvement and agreement on their emphases, there seems to be no reason why check lists cannot be expanded to cover all clinical situations. An important caution lies in the fact that no standardized check list should be used. Each check list must reflect the specific clinical emphases of a specific group of faculty members if it is to work effectively. One point that should be re-emphasized is that a good check list must include opportunities to check whether the instructor has had no opportunity to observe.

One other method of reporting student progress has been described by Stewart and Graham (1968). They describe a *student progress guide* and *visit plan.* The student progress guide consists of eight pages, both sides, divided into rectangles. The first five pages deal with cognitive evaluation, the next two are concerned with the affective domain, and the last page covers psychomotor skills. The guide is readily accessible to instructors and students throughout the clinical experience. The visit plan, prepared by the student, sounds essentially like a variation of a nursing care plan. It enables the instructor to assess the student's progress in data collecting, assessment of health needs, identification of health goals, priority setting, nursing intervention skills, and theoretical background. Again, an important point is that both the instructor and the individual student share the responsibility for evaluating the student's progress.

## SELF-RATINGS AND PEER RATINGS

In describing the use of rating scales and check lists, we have been concentrating on forms and procedures for assessment to be utilized by instructors in the clinical area. Other supplementary methods can greatly enhance the process of evaluation. It should be remembered that we have been emphasizing a system of evaluation that actively involves both the student and the instructor in the learning process. This same principle should apply in the area of assessment and evaluation; i.e. the student must be an active part of the evaluation process.

We have suggested some guidelines for the development and utilization of rating scales and check lists based on clearly stated behavioral objectives. We have stressed that these objectives and evaluation criteria should be clearly communicated to students at the beginning of each clinical sequence, and that students should be given constant, detailed feedback about their progress toward meeting the qualification or successful completion criteria. At the completion of each clinical sequence, and at periodic intervals during the sequence, instructors complete evaluation forms on each student. At the same time, students can be asked to complete the same rating form on themselves independently of the instructor.

At the clinical or final evaluation conference the student can bring in her evaluation form to be compared with and discussed with the instructor. It may be that both agree on current progress and future objectives. Discrepancies, however, need to be examined closely. If an instructor rates an area high or passing, and the student rates herself low or failing, then the instructor may need to deal through counseling with a student with a poor self-concept or unrealistic estimate of her own ability. On the other hand, if the student rates herself high and the instructor rates her low, this has to be examined carefully. It may be that the student's self-appraisal is unrealistic in the face of specific evidence. It may be that the student is correct in her self-appraisal, but that she is giving the wrong signals in her methods of communicating with others. It may also be that the student really can function in a particular area, and that she should be given another opportunity to demonstrate the required skills.

In other words, the dual assessment by the student and the instructor, with each open to change in the light of the conference, can greatly facilitate the effectiveness of the assessment process and the final evaluation conference. It serves to provide more information to both, a result that inevitably will increase the validity of clinical evaluation. Dyer (1971) sums up self-evaluation by stating:

> Self-evaluation by the student should begin with the first course and continue throughout the program. Evaluation devices such as the rat-

ing scale for student self-evaluation may be used. This scale should describe the objectives of the course and should be discussed in detail with the instructor, who makes her evaluation of the student on an identical form and then compares the evaluations.

The same principle may apply to the use of peer ratings. These will be effective only when completed anonymously and with a high level of trust between students and faculty. Systematic peer feedback can be given in a variety of ways, both written and oral. When used properly, it helps to add a third dimension to the evaluation process. We recognize that the final responsibility for evaluation must rest with the faculty. Nevertheless each student has a responsibility to herself, her peers, and the profession she is entering. Therefore she should share in the responsibility for systematic, open, and honest assessment of her own strengths and weaknesses, and those of her classmates with whom she works. Ideally, this same approach could greatly increase the effectiveness of any health sciences team working regularly together. Dyer (1971) again summarizes this point:

> Evaluation by peer group is a new concept to some schools. Nursing students can learn much from observing each other's performance; however, unless this observation, with the aid of a list of behavioral objectives, is planned and discussed thoroughly before it takes place and in a constructive manner afterwards, such an evaluation can be catastrophic. . . . The instructor can also evaluate the observation skills of the observer.

## EVALUATION CONFERENCES

The progress reports or final evaluation conferences are a vitally important part of successful and educationally sound clinical evaluation. These conferences need to be carefully planned for by both the student and the instructor. Both must have a clear understanding of the purpose of the conference in advance. Ideally, it is to provide a time for the sharing of information about the student's progress in as nonthreatening an atmosphere as possible. Both should have the opportunity to gather whatever information is necessary to bring to the conference.

Cobb, Rose, and Schuman (1965) reported the results of a faculty debate on the pros and cons of conducting individual clinical conferences. Some of the negative reasons given were the investment of time needed, and the unpleasantness of having to debate grades with students. The majority concluded that if time permits, frequent individual conferences should be held with students. In many respects, this is a poor debate with a poor conclusion. It is not a question as to whether or not time permits. It is essential for student-faculty communication that an open, valid, fair, and consistent evaluation system be developed, maintained, and safeguarded. Without individual conferences at regular intervals, evaluation tends to become biased and autocratic, for the instructor never needs to defend her evaluations.

Calamari (1968) reports a simple questionnaire study that sums up many of the desirable aspects of a good evaluation conference. Students were asked to state their feelings about their final evaluation conferences. The results included the following points:

1. Students felt that it was important to know the objectives and requirements of the clinical experience before it began.

2. Students preferred to have anecdotal and similar material available to them at all times during the clinical experience to review.

3. Students preferred frequent contact with and feedback from their clinical instructors.

4. Students wanted clinical conferences conducted in privacy and with sufficient time to talk.

5. Students wanted the freedom and opportunity to discuss their feelings about the evaluation and the conclusions drawn.

6. Students felt that the atmosphere should be relaxed and open, preferably in another place than a faculty office.

What the students are at least partially saying is that they want constant feedback from their instructor as to how she thinks they are meeting the objectives, rather than just comments at the final evaluation conference. A good conference can be positively anticipated by both students and faculty if the guidelines suggested above are followed.

Clinical evaluation has frequently been a difficult and frustrating experience for both faculty members and students. The guidelines suggested in this chapter will not eliminate all problems, but they should serve to make clinical evaluation a valuable, constructive, ongoing part of the total educational experience.

## BIBLIOGRAPHY

### Part 2

Ahmann, J. Stanley, and Glock, Marion D.: *Evaluating Pupil Growth*. Boston, Allyn and Bacon, Inc., 1963.

Anastasi, Anne: *Psychological Testing*. 3rd ed. New York, Macmillian Company, 1970.

Anderson, Diann M.: Performance Evaluation of Nursing Students. *Nursing Outlook*, Vol. 16, No. 6, 1968, pp. 56–58.

Armstrong, Robert, J., Cornell, Terry D., Kraner, Robert B., and Roberson, Wayne E.: *The Development and Evaluation of Behavioral Objectives*. Worthington, Ohio, Charles A. Jones Publishing Company, 1970.

Barrett, Evelyn R., and Irion, Lou Ann: Advantages and Disadvantages of Nongrading. *Nursing Outlook*, Vol. 18, No. 4, 1970, pp. 40–41.

Berzon, Faye Clark: Use of Extended Care Facility for Beginning Students. *Nursing Outlook*, Vol. 18, No. 11, 1970, pp. 44–46.

Bitzer, Maryann: Clinical Nursing Instruction Via the Plato Simulated Laboratory. *Nursing Research*, Vol. 15, No. 2, Spring, 1966, pp. 144–150.

Blakeney, Hazel Elizabeth: Evaluation of Student Achievement in Associate Degree Nursing Programs, Unpublished Doctoral Dissertation, Columbia University, 1967.

Bloom, Benjamin S. (Ed.): *Taxonomy of Educational Objectives: The Classification of Educational Goals. Handbook I, Cognitive Domain*. New York, Longmans, Green, and Co., 1956.

Bohan, Sister Kathleen Mary: Performance Relationship: Nursing Student to Professional

Nurse. Unpublished Doctoral Dissertation, Catholic University of America, Vol. 27-A, 1966.

Brester, Mary, Loews, Grace, Carozza, Virginia J., and Bernard, Margaret C.; Evaluating Nursing Students. *American Journal of Nursing*, Vol. 62, No. 5, 1962, pp. 117–119.

Calamari, Sister Dolores: Factors That Influence Evaluation Conferences in Clinical Experience. *Journal of Nursing Education*, Vol. 7, No. 4, 1968, pp. 11–14.

Cautela, Joseph R.: Low Probability Hypothesis. *Personnel and Guidance Journal*, Vol. 42, No. 1, 1964, pp. 670–673.

Cobb, Marguerite, Rose, Patricia, and Schuman, Delores: The Pros and Cons of Formal Education Conferences: A Faculty Debate. *Nursing Forum*, Vol. 4, No. 4, 1965, pp. 67–75.

Collins, Harold W., Johnson, John, and Johnson, James A.: *Educational Measurement and Evaluation: A Work Text*. Glenview, Ill., Scott, Foresman and Co., 1969.

Cronbach, Lee J.: *Essentials of Psychological Testing*. 3rd. ed. New York, Harper & Bros., 1967.

Crowley, Dorothy: Clinical Diaries: A Part of the Teaching Learning Process. *Journal of Nursing Education*, Vol. 4, No. 4, 1965, pp. 19–21.

Curriculum Sub-Committee on Rating Scales, University of Arizona: Let's Examine—The Method of Developing Performance Rating Scales. *Nursing Outlook*, Vol. 18, No. 10, 1970, p. 57.

David, Frederick B.: *Item-Analysis Data: Their Computation, Interpretation, and Use in Test Construction*. Cambridge, Harvard University, Harvard Education Papers, Number 2, 1964.

Downie, N. M.: *Fundamentals of Measurement: Techniques and Practices*. New York, Oxford Union Press, 1967.

Dunn, Margaret A.: Development of an Instrument to Measure Nursing Performance. *Nursing Research*, Vol. 19, No. 6, 1970, pp. 502–510.

Durham, R. C.: How to Evaluate Nursing Performance. *Nursing Research*, Vol. 19, No. 6, 1970, p. 552.

Dyer, Marilyn: *Keeping on Course*. Report of the 1970 Regional Workshops of the Council of Diploma Programs. New York, National League of Nursing, 1971.

Ebel, Robert L.: Procedures for the Analysis of Classroom Tests. *Educational and Psychological Measurement*, Vol. 14, Summer, 1954, pp. 352–364.

Ebel, Robert L.: *Nursing Educational Achievement*, Englewood Cliffs, N.J. Prentice-Hall, 1965.

Edwards, Allen L.: *Statistical Methods for the Behavioral Science*. New York, Rinehard & Co., 1954.

Esbensen, Thorwald: *Working with Individualized Instruction: The Duluth Experience*. Belmont, Calif., Fearon Publishers, 1968.

Ferguson, George A.: *Statistical Analysis in Psychology and Education*. New York, McGraw-Hill Book Company, Inc., 1959.

Fivars, Grace, and Gosnell, Doris: *Nursing Evaluation: The Problem and the Process*. New York, Macmillan Company, 1966.

Frejlach, Grace, and Corcoran, Sheila: Measuring Clinical Performance. *Nursing Outlook*, Vol. 19, No. 4, 1971, pp. 270–271.

Furst, E. J.: *Constructing Evaluation Instruments*. New York, Longmans, Green and Co., 1958.

Galeener, Janet: Providing More Meaningful Clinical Experiences Through Group or Multiple Student Assignment. *Journal of Nursing Education*, Vol. 5, No. 2, 1966, pp. 29–31.

Gerchberg, Louise Rozario: *An Observational Method for Evaluating the Performance of Nursing Students in Clinical Situations*. New York, National League for Nursing, 1962.

Green, John, A.: *Introduction to Measurement and Evaluation*. New York, Mead and Co., 1940.

Hamm, Betty H., and Hartsfield, Sandra L.: Motivation Influencing Students in Psychiatric Nursing. *Nursing Research*, Vol. 19, No. 1, 1970, pp. 79–81.

Hazeltine, Louise S., and Zetz, Leonard: Evaluating Clinical Performance. *Nursing Outlook*, Vol. 12, No. 8, 1964, pp. 33–35.

Kemp, Jerrold, B.: *Instructional Design*. Richmond, Calif., Fearon Publishers, 1971.

Klausmeier, Herbert J.: *Learning and Human Abilities*. New York, Harper & Brothers, 1961.

Komorita, Nori I.: Student Opinions Towards Methods of Guidance and Evaluation in Clinical Nursing. *Nursing Research*, Vol. 14, No. 2, Spring, 1965, pp. 163–167.

Kramer, Marlene: Does Teacher Really Know Best? *Journal of Nursing Education*, Vol. 6, No. 1, 1967, pp. 3–11, 24–27.

Krathwohl, D. R. (Ed.): *Taxonomy of Educational Objectives: The Classification of Educational Goals. Handbook II, Affective Domain*. New York, Longmans, Green and Co., 1965.

Lenz, Elizabeth, and Bauer, Edith Clark: An Integrated Nursing Care Study. *Nursing Out-look,* Vol. 18, No. 7, 1970, pp. 36–37.

Lyman, H. B.: *Test Scores and What They Mean.* Englewood Cliffs, N.J., Prentice-Hall, Inc., 1963.

McCaffery, Margo: What Is the Student Teaching in the Clinical Laboratory? *Journal of Nursing Education,* Vol. 7, No. 4, 1968, pp. 3–10.

Mager, Robert, R.: *Preparing Instructional Objectives.* Palo Alto, Calif., Fearon Publishers, 1962.

Moritz, Derry, and Sexton, Dorothy: Evaluation: A Suggested Method for Appraising Quality. *Journal of Nursing Education,* Vol. 9, No. 1, 1970, pp. 17–34.

Murphy, Juanita: The Nub of the Learning Process. *American Journal of Nursing,* Vol. 71, No. 2, February, 1971, pp. 306–310.

Nehren, J., and Batey, M.: Process Recording. *Nursing Forum,* Vol. 2, No. 2, 1963, pp. 65–73.

Odell, C. W.: Marks and Marking System; in W. S. Monroe (Ed.): *Encyclopedia of Educational Research.* New York, Macmillan Company, 1950.

Ortelt, Judith: The Development of a Scale for Rating Clinical Performance. *Journal of Nursing Education,* Vol. 5, No. 1, 1966, pp. 15–17.

O'Shea, Helen Spustek: A Guide to Evaluation of Clinical Performance. *American Journal of Nursing,* Vol. 67, No. 9, Sept., 1967, pp. 1877–1879.

Palmer, Mary Ellen: *Self Evaluation of Nursing Performance Based on Clinical Practice Objectives.* Boston, Boston University Press, 1962.

Palmer, Mary Ellen: Our Students Write Their Own Behavioral Anecdotes. *Nursing Outlook,* Vol. II, No. 3, 1963.

Palmer, Mary Ellen: Self-Evaluation of Clinical Performance. *Nursing Outlook,* Vol. 15, No. 11, 1967, pp. 63–65.

Redman, Barbara K.: Clinical Nursing Instructors' Perception of Students' Attitudes Toward Selected Interpersonal Relationship. Unpublished Doctoral Dissertation, University of Minnesota, Vol. 26, No. 1, 1964, pp. 59–63.

Redman, Barbara K.: Nursing Teacher Perceptiveness of Student Attitudes. *Nursing Research,* Vol. 17, No. 5, 1968, p. 375.

Rines, Alice R.: *Evaluating Student Progress in Learning the Practice of Nursing.* New York, Bureau of Publication, Teachers College, Columbia University, 1963.

Schultz, Frances K.: Evaluation: Signpost of Judgment. *Nursing Outlook,* Vol. 12, No. 9, 1964, pp. 57–58.

Schwier, Mildred, and Davidson, E. Rita: *Improving Test Construction.* (League Exchange No 59.) New York, National League for Nursing, 1962.

Seivwright, Mary Jane: The Expectations of Baccalaureate Nursing Students Concerning Their Clinical Experience in Public Health Nursing. Unpublished Doctoral Dissertation, Columbia University, Vol. 30-B, 1968.

Shields, Mary R.: *The Construction and Use of Teacher-Made Tests.* 2nd ed. (Use of Tests in Schools of Nursing, Pamphlet No. 5.) New York, National League for Nursing, 1965.

Shield, Mary: Let's Examine—A Scoring Problem in Performance Assessment. *Nursing Outlook,* Vol. 16, No. 8, 1968, pp. 61–62.

Silvern, Leonard C.: *System Engineering of Education I; The Evolution of System Thinking in Education.* Los Angeles, Educational and Training Consultants Co., 1968.

Simpson, June: The Walk-Around Laboratory Practical Examination in Evaluative Clinical Nursing Skills. *Journal of Nursing Education,* Vol. 6, No. 4, 1967, pp. 23–26.

Slater, Doris: *The Slater Nursing Competencies Rating Scale.* Detroit, Mich., Wayne State University College of Nursing, Mimeographed, 1967.

Smeltzer, C. H.: *Psychological Evaluations in Nursing Education.* New York, Macmillan Company, 1965.

Smith, Kathryn Muriel: Discrepancies in the Value Climate of Nursing Students: A Comparison of Head Nurses and Nursing Educators. *Nursing Research,* Vol. 14, No. 7, Summer, 1965, pp. 196–197.

Smith, Virginia Whitmore: I Can't Believe I Said That! *Nursing Outlook,* Vol. 18, No. 5, 1970, pp. 50, 51.

Staff of NLN Test Services. Let's Examine—This Matter of Guessing. *Nursing Outlook,* Vol. 10, No. 3, 1962, p. 185.

Staff of NLN Test Construction Unit: Let's Examine—Behavior. *Nursing Outlook,* Vol. 12, No. 5, 1964, p. 65.

Stevens, Delphie: A Tool For Evaluating Clinical Performance. *American Journal of Nursing*, Vol. 70, No. 6, June, 1970, pp. 1308–1310.

Stevens, S. S.: Mathematics, Measurement, and Psycho Physics; In S. S. Stevens (Ed.): *Handbook of Experimental Psychology*. New York, John Wiley & Sons, 1951.

Stewart, Ruth, and Graham, Josephine L.: Evaluation Tools in Public Health Nursing Education. *Nursing Outlook*, Vol. 16, No. 3, 1968, pp. 50–51.

Tadlock, Jane E.: Student Participation in Evaluating Clinical Skills. *Journal of Nursing Education*, Vol. 3, No. 4, 1964, pp. 5–7, 20.

Thorndike, Robert L., and Hagen, Elizabeth: *Measurement and Evaluation in Psychology and Education*. 3rd. ed. New York, John Wiley & Sons, 1969.

Torgerson, Warren, S.: *Theory and Methods of Scaling*. New York, John Wiley & Sons., Inc., 1965.

Tornyay, Rheba: Measuring Problem Solving Skills by Means of the Simulated Clinical Nursing Problem Test. *Journal of Nursing Education*, Vol. 7, No. 3, 1968, pp. 3–8, 34–35.

Treece, Eleanor: Students' Opinions Concerning Patient Selection for Clinical Practice. *Journal of Nursing Education*, Vol. 8, No. 2, 1969, pp. 17–21, 24–25.

Treece, Eleanor: *Level of Objectives—Development and Use in Curriculum*. New York, National League of Nursing, 1970.

Westley, Bruce H., and Hornback, May: An Experimental Study of the Use of Television in Teaching Basic Nursing Skills. *Nursing Research*, Vol. 13, No. 3, Summer, 1964, pp. 205–209.

Wood, Dorothy Adkins: *Test Construction*. Columbus, Ohio, Charles Merrill, 1961.

Zasowska, Sister Mary Aloiseanne: A Descriptive Survey of Significant Factors in the Clinical Laboratory Experience in Baccalaureate Education for Nursing. Unpublished Doctoral Dissertation, Columbia University, Vol. 28-B, 1967.

Part 3

# Student Development

# Chapter 11

# Standardized Tests

In Part 2 of this book we analyzed the process of measurement and evaluation in the classroom and clinical areas of nursing education. We concentrated particularly on assessment procedures developed and used within each school of nursing by faculty members. These are important, and should represent the core of the ongoing evaluation process from admission to graduation. In addition, attention needs to be given to the use of standardized tests in nursing education, for they can provide valuable supplements both to the in-school evaluation criteria and the ongoing guidance and counseling program. By standardized tests, we refer to nationally developed paper-and-pencil tests that allow the faculty within a particular school to compare its students with others on local and national levels.

Standardized tests can be and are used for a variety of purposes within nursing education. These may be listed as follows:

   a. Prediction tests
   b. Pre-entrance tests
   c. Placement tests
   d. Achievement tests
   e. Licensure examinations
   f. Personality tests
   g. Tests for guidance and self-understanding.

Each of these groups represents areas in which standardized tests, when used properly, can provide valuable additional information to educational programming and the development of student services. In almost every situation the use of standardized instruments should depend on the availability of qualified people to interpret the results in ways designed to help students succeed in achieving the goals of nursing education. It must be emphasized from the outset that standardized tests are not panaceas for the problems in nursing education; they are not foolproof predictors of anything; and they are beset with problems arising from the misuse of results in ways which are educationally and psychologically unsound. It should be clear that standardized tests are discussed throughout this book with the purpose of guidance and counseling in mind, rather than as bases for decisions.

## PRE-ENTRANCE TESTS

In discussing pre-entrance tests we are concerned with the nationally standardized tests used widely by schools of nursing to help them make decisions about admission. We will discuss in the next chapter the wide variety of factors in current efforts to predict success in schools of nursing. At this point we are primarily concerned with the NLN Pre-Nursing and Guidance Examination. It is recognized that many schools of nursing utilize the American College Test (ACT) prepared by Science Research Associates of Chicago, or the College Entrance Examination Boards (CEEB) prepared by the Educational Testing Service of Princeton, N. J., to help in the determination of admission eligibility.

The NLN Pre-Nursing and Guidance Examination was originally developed by the National League for Nursing for possible use as a selection and guidance tool by nursing educators. The original PNG comprised five tests from which eight test scores and a composite score were obtained. These included the Test of Academic Aptitude, which provided a verbal, quantitative, and total score; the Reading Comprehension Test, which provided speed and level of comprehension scores; the Mathematics Test; the Natural Sciences Achievement Test; and the Social Studies Achievement Test. In 1970 a report on the NLN PNG was issued based on a study sample of 12,552 students who entered 314 schools of nursing. The sample included 241 students entering seven AD programs, and the remaining 11,671 entering 288 diploma programs. Several of the generalizations and conclusions reached are worth commenting on here.

1. PNG scores of entrants exceeded those of applicants. This is a meaningless generalization that is hardly surprising. Since many schools use the PNG as a selection tool, and admit those with the best scores, it logically figures that those who entered would probably have significantly better PNG scores than those who were rejected. In other words, those who entered were a select group from those students who applied.

2. At each stage of the educational program, PNG scores of students who remained exceeded those of students who withdrew for classroom or clinical failure. This could be an important point. If the difference in scores was significant, then the results would seem to indicate that the PNG could be used to predict academic success and failure. Nevertheless the data presented fail to report on significance, so that conclusions must be interpreted with caution.

3. Each of the tests on the PNG correlated significantly with each of the tests on the State Boards, and the PNG as a whole correlated significantly with performance on the State Boards as a whole. This may indicate nothing more than that the tests measure similar things. Also, the confounding factor is the unknown extent to which faculty members are governed by the PNG scores and the State Board emphases in planning their teaching.

In 1971 the NLN PNG was completely revised. The new battery is composed of four tests instead of the previous five. The Mathematics Test is no longer administered. The Academic Aptitude Test, as before, measures basic verbal and mathematical abilities. Three scores are derived from the Academic Aptitude Test: verbal, quantitative, and a total score. The verbal score can be a useful indicator of general ability, and can provide information about applicants who need individual attention and remedial work in order to succeed in the nursing program. The quantitative score is also helpful in identifying applicants who could profit from re-medial instruction, since it involves a minimum of cultural influence.

The new reading test provides one score, based on the applicant's ability to read and understand. The new science test evaluates the applicant's ability to identify and define scientific problems, interpret data, and perform symbolic and quantitative reasoning. The social studies test score measures ability to understand and interpret materials such as maps, graphs, historical documents, and editorials. A composite score is also reported, but there seems to be little current evidence warranting its use for anything.

The Revised Pre-Nursing and Guidance Examination is still too new to evaluate its effectiveness as a diagnostic tool. The first set of norms will not be available until some time in the latter half of 1972. Nevertheless the new test does stress one important point. The NLN emphasizes that the focus on the use of preadmissions tests such as the PNG be for guidance and placement purposes rather than for selection. For this it is essential that programs and resources be made available for tutorial and remedial assistance to applicants who might otherwise be rejected or fail.

The important thing to remember here is that the revised PNG, or, for that matter, the ACT and the CEEB, are useful guides rather telling us more about the students who come to us than serving as perfect predictors which should be interpreted rigidly in determining who shall come in and who shall stay out. If students have already taken the ACT or the Scholastic Aptitude Test (SAT) of the CEEB, there is a real question as to the value of requiring them to take the PNG in addition. There seems to be little evidence that the PNG measures something unique which is not measured on either the ACT or the SAT. Therefore why require students to take an additional test? Each school of nursing must analyze what, if anything, the PNG provides that is not already available in school records or in performance on the ACT or the SAT.

For example, Miller et al. (1968) reported that the SAT verbal score was one of six variables that proved to be the most efficient in predicting the State Board scores and the chances of failure on each of the five SBE tests. Ledbetter (1968) concluded that the ACT, the NLN Achievement Tests, and the State Board subtests appear to measure a degree of common factors. In addition, scores on the ACT appear to be consistent with students' achievement, as indicated by their cumulative grade point averages, during the total educational program.

The point is that the PNG should not be used merely because it happens to be available. If a student has previously taken other tests, then the faculty needs to determine what, if any, unique information is provided by the PNG. For example, Muhlencamp (1971) found that the most significant predictor of State Board scores was the students' grade point average. Considering the amount of information normally available on each applicant, and considering the availability of the ACT and the CEEB, there seems to be a valid question as to the rationale for the existence and use of the PNG, particularly in AD and baccalaureate programs. With the rapid movement of nursing education into educational settings, with the trend for high school students who wish to go on for further education to take either the ACT or the CEEB, and with the current practice of two-year and four-year colleges requiring scores on the ACT or the SAT for admission, it may be time to consider phasing out the PNG as superfluous for nursing education. Diploma schools may wish to consider switching to either the ACT or the SAT, unless they have found specific benefits that can be gained from the PNG. Certainly more research is needed in this area, accompanied by some long-range planning.

In examining the use of preadmission tests, we must recognize the existence of cultural bias in all the existing tests. Much has been written in books and journals about the cultural bias which is an inherent characteristic of practically all standardized tests in current use. By the term "cultural bias" we mean the use of language and concepts that are typically understood by the white, middle-class, American student, but which penalize the culturally different student with a different set of values, understandings, and vocabulary, such as the black, the Puerto Rican, the Indian, the Chicano, and others. The problems created by culturally biased tests are receiving increasing attention in education and industry—in fact, in all segments of society currently using standardized tests.

Tests in current use for admission into higher education, including the PNG, are culturally biased in terms of vocabulary, reading level, and content. With the current emphasis in nursing education upon recruitment of the culturally different, tests such as the PNG unnecessarily handicap a prospective student. Faculty members may feel that they recognize the problems of cultural bias, and thus use the tests only as guidance tools rather than as selection devices. In too many cases, however, faculty members fail to understand what cultural bias means, and what potentially devastating effects the use of culturally biased tests may have on students.

There are several reasons why culturally biased tests remain a problem even with sophisticated faculty members. First, some faculty members tend to label students on the basis of tests scores. Even if scores are not used as a barrier to admission, a student with high scores tends to be viewed positively by the faculty, and a student with low scores is viewed as a likely failure. This almost inevitably contributes to a self-fulfilling prophecy on the part of the faculty—we expect the student to fail, and she does. Second, students themselves begin to doubt their own ability and self-worth when they do poorly on standardized tests. Again, the self-fulfilling prophecy begins to be true, and students pay the price for a test that was of debatable validity for use with them. In general, faculty members need to re-examine seriously the use of any standardized test as a screening tool. Is what we gain worth the price of what we lose in student anxiety, attitudes, and discouragement? Are preadmission tests really necessary, or can we obtain the information we need through high school performance, recommendations, and interviews? Cannot we rest our decisions and programs on professional judgment without relying on the false security of tests as predictive or selective devices? Certainly this is an area of nursing education that needs to be carefully researched.

## PLACEMENT TESTS

One problem that has plagued nursing educators is the question of systematic procedures for admitting graduates of AD and diploma programs into baccalaureate programs in nursing. The same problem occurs in admitting diploma graduates into AD programs, and LPN'S into any of the three main kinds of nursing schools. At one time some colleges such as Teachers College, Columbia University, gave two years' automatic credit to any graduate of a diploma program. But as time went by the trend seemed to shift away from automatic credit toward a more systematic way of evaluating the level of each applicant. This occurred as colleges found that graduate nurses had widely varying skills and knowledge, resulting from the wide variance in the quality of the nursing program from which they graduated. In an apparent effort to upgrade the profession of nursing, the new directions seemed to fall into two groups, the use of nationally standardized tests for proper placement, and locally developed procedures.

In 1965 the NLN reported on the progressive development of the Graduate Nurse Examination (GNE) over a 30-year period. By that time between 5000 and 6000 students were taking the test yearly. The Steering Committee of the Department of Baccalaureate and Higher Degree Programs of the NLN felt that the GNE could be used for placement testing of graduates from other programs. In 1969 the NLN reported on the increasing use of proficiency examinations in admitting registered nurses to baccalaureate programs. It was felt that the faculty within each school had to examine the use of such tests in relation to their course and program objectives. Perhaps the best source for an overview of this area is provided by the annotated bibliography issued by the NLN in October, 1969, dealing with challenge examinations and their particular focus on the registered nurse entering a baccalaureate program.

Reviewing several of the studies reported by the NLN, Malkin (1966) emphasized the need for adequate counseling for diploma and AD graduates who wish to enter baccalaureate programs. She expressed particular concern over provisions for adequate guidance and support for those who fail challenge examinations. The University of Arizona School of Nursing reported in 1969 that they allow up to 60 units of credit to be challenged for credit by examination. In addition to nationally standardized tests such as the GNE, they reported the use of teacher-made objective, essay, and performance tests. There is no penalty for failing, and actual course credit is given the successful challenger. Katzell (1970) added several points to those previously mentioned. She suggests that consideration be given to the use of NLN achievement tests for evaluating the background and skills of practical nurses seeking admission to an AD or baccalaureate program. She emphasizes that systematic observation of clinical performance in the clinical area should also be conducted. She advocates the use of standardized tests instead of teacher-made tests. Her last point is somewhat debatable. Although it will be a more objective method, it assumes that the course and program objectives within a college are the same as the objectives emphasized on the nationally standardized tests.

In general, there seems to be consensus as to the use of a variety of challenge procedures for graduate nurses applying to baccalaureate programs. Each school of nursing must test out and constantly review the procedures that work best within the particular school. Emphasis must be placed upon some method of assessing the student's ability to meet the levels of minimal competency established within each course in the baccalaureate program. Although standardized tests such as the GNE may be used, much more research is needed to support such a practice. In order to assess legitimately the student's ability to meet all the local objectives, it may be desirable to place the greatest emphasis on teacher-made tests within the particular school along with systematic clinical evaluation in order to determine the proper placement for an individual student.

There is another way in which placement examinations are applied, and this is the use of standardized tests to predict success in particular course sequences. Through successful prediction, early identification can be made of those who have a high potential for failure so that provision can be made for prior remedial work and concurrent tutorial assistance. Mancott (1969) reports the use of one such method in an AD program. A study was made of 112 second-year students to assess the validity of two measures in the prediction of success in a general chemistry course. The two predictors were the Lorge-Thorndike Intelligence Test, Verbal and Non-verbal Batteries, Level 5, Form A. Of the 51 students who failed the course, 41 had nonverbal IQ's below the class mean of 102.3. A second study by Mancott in 1970 reinforced the earlier study. This time, 30 of the 47 students who failed the course had nonverbal IQ's below the class mean of 102.5. He also found that older students seem to have the most difficulty in coping with abstract concepts, abstract analogies, and number concepts.

Placement tests as predictive tools should be used primarily for guidance and counseling. The use of cut-off scores to determine admission or placement is an educationally unsound practice. Such use implies much greater validity than any test warrants, and ignores sound measurement principles such as the standard error of measurement. Placement tests can, however, be useful as diagnostic tools to assist in the educational programming for individual students when used along with other methods of evaluation.

## ACHIEVEMENT TESTS

In Chapter 9 we discussed the use of teacher-made tests to measure knowledge and skills in the classroom and academic areas. We also mentioned that such tests could be useful as diagnostic tools indicating areas of weakness. Standardized achievement tests such as the NLN Achievement Tests can also be useful in fulfilling a diagnostic function. At present the NLN Achievement Tests are not used in all schools of nursing, although their use is common enough to warrant a closer look.

The NLN Achievement Tests are comprehensive tests designed to provide broader coverage of a field and to require greater depth and breadth of understanding. As the NLN pointed out in 1962, the Achievement Tests should not be used to dictate course content, although faculty members may wish to reconsider material that they are deleting from a course while others in the field think it important. The comment made by the NLN at that time was that the national tests should not include new and untried ideas. A year later the NLN Test Services began to question whether one series of standardized achievement tests was equally suitable for all kinds of programs in nursing education. In 1963 the idea was presented that the NLN Achievement Tests may help in evaluating students' ability to use previously learned facts and principles as a basis for identifying and solving new nursing problems. It was felt that one way of doing this was to administer tests which present nursing situations that are unfamiliar to the students. For example, in 1965 the NLN traced the development of one achievement test, the psychiatric nursing test, as it evolved through the years. Earlier tests pertained to the identification of specific diseases, symptoms, and awareness of the guardianship role of nurses. In the 1950's test questions concentrated on the use of nondirective replies, and methods of helping patients with reality. By the 1960's some of the old was retained, but the test now emphasized the active role of the nurse in seeking data and in talking to patients about their concerns and feelings. This history of change reflects the different emphases seen over the years in the NLN Achievement Tests.

In 1966 the 18-month to two-year procedure followed in developing an NLN Achievement Test was described, from the initial determination of need to the final publication and development of norms. In the same year, procedures for preparing students to take the NLN Achievement Tests were described. One interesting comment made at this time was that students' attitudes toward the NLN Achievement Tests frequently reflect the attitudes of the faculty; i.e. if the faculty downgrade the value of the tests, then students will do the same.

Thus we can see the development of the national testing program over the years to the point at which the NLN Achievement Tests today are in relatively common use. Yet the question needs to be raised as to the appropriateness of much of the current usage. Several factors need to be examined. First, in many cases, faculty members may find themselves teaching for the test. Curricular emphases tend to become identical with the emphases in the test being used. Since the national tests as described by the NLN attempt to steer away from new and untried ideas, the result too often may be an emphasis on and assessment of safe ideas, rather than on new and creative approaches.

Second, the tests are sometimes used for curricular evaluation. At times this may be accompanied by faculty evaluation. Both these practices are unsound. The more this is done, the more faculty members will tend to teach for the tests. More importantly, such practices tend to stifle teaching creativity, and foster conformity to national norms. The tests cease to become a tool, and become an objective to be reached.

Third, the question needs to be asked as to the purpose behind the use of the NLN Achievement Tests. Why are they administered? Some of the reasons stated include the following: to measure learning in an area, to predict results on the State Boards, to compare students with others on a local or national level, and to give students practice in taking standardized tests.

None of these reasons has built-in validity. The best way to measure learning in a particular area is through classroom and clinical evaluation procedures developed by the faculty members within the particular school that are designed to represent the emphases within that school. Predicting results on the State Boards may be fine if the prime objective of nursing education is to prepare students for the State Boards. But even if this were a primary goal, studies have indicated that the best predictor is still course grades. Comparing students with those in other schools is at best an academic exercise in futility; it serves little purpose. All schools are not at the same level; instructors have different levels of preparation; and curricular emphases will differ.

Our primary objective is to help each student develop to her full capacity. It is irrelevant to compare her with others as long as she at least meets the level of minimal competency established within a school. Giving students practice in taking standardized tests may be a desirable guidance function, but it is definitely not a function of evaluation. Finally, the NLN Achievement Tests have at times been used as final examinations within particular schools. No national test can ever legitimately serve this function unless the objectives within a school of nursing are identical with the curricular emphases found on the tests. It is highly unlikely that this will occur in any school with a competent creative faculty.

Nevertheless the NLN Achievement Tests may have a useful function. The faculty of a particular school must first develop its own curriculum and specific course objectives. The entire educational program should be developed as a result of the best thinking of the faculty. After this has been done the NLN tests may be used as diagnostic tools. Since the NLN Achievement Tests have similar emphases as the State Boards, students can be helped to overcome deficiencies that they will later have to demonstrate on the State Boards. This diagnostic and remedial function should, however, not be done at the expense of the normal, ongoing educational program. Recognizing that the State Boards are currently a hurdle for students to overcome at the end of training, anything we can do to help students meet this hurdle easily may be useful.

A more desirable model for a standardized test was reported by Metz (1964). She developed and validated a standardized test to measure achievement of the cognitive aspects of objectives of efficient body movement for nursing students. She reported the original development in the state of Washington, and the final version which was given to 341 students in selected state-accredited schools of nursing in five Western regional states excluding Washington. The standardization procedures she followed provided useful guidelines for others to follow. Thus the best general rule of thumb is that achievement tests are best developed on the local level. Nationally standardized achievement tests should be used with great caution, if at all, and then only after constant study and review by the faculty within each school. It would seem that the NLN could perhaps provide a valuable service as a resource to help local schools develop their own tests on sound measurement principles.

# PREDICTION OF STATE BOARD SCORES

Students learn quickly upon entering a school of nursing that ultimately they will be required to take State Board examinations to be licensed as registered nurses after graduation from the school. Thereafter this becomes a concern that never really is resolved until the students are successful on the State Boards. Faculty members are equally aware of the State Boards, and are concerned about getting their students ready for them. With this concern ever in mind, it is not surprising that constant efforts have been made to predict performance on the State Boards, so that those who are predicted to be unsuccessful can receive extra tutorial and remedial assistance to upgrade their skills and competencies.

Brandt et al. (1966) studied the relations between therapy and practice grades within the curriculum and results on the NLN Achievement Tests and success on the State Board Test Pool Examination (SBE). They concluded that grades received in nursing therapy courses, and scores on the Natural Science, Social Science, and NLN Basic Medical-Surgical Achievement Test have a positive correlation with the SBE, and may be useful in predicting performance. Baldwin et al. (1968) found somewhat different results. They found a positive correlation between NLN Achievement Tests and SBE scores, but no significant correlation between theory grades and SBE scores. They also found that students developed a more positive attitude toward the NLN Achievement Tests as diagnostic tools, once they were shown the relation between the tests and SBE scores.

Miller et al. (1968) looked at the problems of prediction on a broader base. They found six variables that were most efficient in predicting SBE scores. These were the SAT verbal score, the educational level of the student's father, the student's age in months upon admission, high school graduation rank in class, the number of college credits completed before entering the nursing program, and the overall grade point average at the end of the nursing program. These six variables were the result of a multiple regression equation to find the best possible predictors.

Ledbetter (1968) studied the relation between the ACT, the NLN Achievement Tests, and the SBE, and found that all three seemed to measure a degree of common factors. She reports further that the subtests of the NLN Achievement Test and the SBE appear to measure common elements within each test as well as between the two tests. She found that scores of nursing students on the ACT, the NLN Graduate Nurse Examination subtest, the NLN Achievement Tests, and the SBE subtests are all consistent with the students' achievement during the total educational program as indicated by their cumulative grade point averages. Most importantly, however, she found that the achievement of nursing students on the NLN Achievement Tests and the SBE subtests generally differs from their performance as determined by the clinical departmental faculty members within the educational program. If we feel that evaluation of students in the clinical area is of prime importance, then this last point would seem to indicate a significant weakness in both tests. The alternative point of view, i.e. that the clinical judgment of the faculty is less valid than the test results, hardly seems tenable. There obviously seems to be a strong need for additional research to verify Ledbetter's results.

The NLN reported in 1970 that the best achievement test predictors of performance on the licensing examination for students in baccalaureate and diploma programs were the three medical-surgical nursing achievement tests. There were highly significant correlations with all nine of the achievement tests. There were too few in the associate degree programs for meaningful results at that time. The NLN concluded that test scores on achievement tests are indicative of the performance which may be expected on State Board examinations. This is not surprising, since, as Ledbetter demonstrated, they apparently are measuring essentially the same things. Nevertheless the NLN Achievement Tests can still be used diagnostically.

Papcam (1971) studied a group of students who graduated from an AD program, 91.3 per cent of whom passed the SBE on the first testing. She found that the best predictor of each of the five tests in the SBE was the NLN Comprehensive Achievement Test in Maternal and Child Nursing, Form 658. The Medical Nursing test of the SBE produced the lowest correlation with total scores on the achievement tests.

In general, the results of the foregoing studies are not too unusual. The pattern seems to indicate a good predictive relation between the NLN Achievement Tests and scores on the SBE. The most significant point was the one reported by Ledbetter; i.e. scores on both the NLN Achievement Tests and the SBE seem to have little relation to clinical evaluations. Although this result occurred in only one study, if it represents a general trend in nursing education, then it would seem to reflect the principal weakness in the SBE. Keeping this last point in mind, let's look a little more closely at the SBE.

## STATE BOARD LICENSURE EXAMINATIONS

Prior to 1942, state boards of nursing prepared their own examinations. As a result there were wide variances in the material covered. The objectives of the *Curriculum Guide for Schools of Nursing* were utilized in building the first tests. Originally there were 13 tests, which were later reduced to the current five. In 1962 the staff of the NLN Test Service reported on the rationale behind the SBE. They stated that safety of practice cannot be dissociated from effectiveness of practice, and that the only way to test for application of knowledge is to present the examinee with a situation that is in some way new.

This philosophy was restated in 1963 when it was indicated that the majority of state boards of nursing and NLN Test Services believe that State Board examinations ensure that successful candidates know enough that their nursing practice will not be unsafe or ineffective. Again, in 1965, it was stated that licensure examinations have as their goal the protection of the public, and that the specific purpose is to make certain that each candidate has at least a certain minimum acceptable amount of nursing knowledge. Thus we have the consistently stated position that

State Board examinations are designed to measure the student's ability to provide safe, competent nursing care. There seems to be an unfortunate connotation to the foregoing emphases; i.e. trust cannot be placed on the faculty within a particular school to judge the competency of the students graduating from that school.

Unfortunately it does not seem as if the SBE really meets the purpose for which is was created. Although one must be careful about generalizing too much from one report, the Ledbetter study clearly pointed up the seeming lack of relation between clinical evaluation and SBE scores. Therefore it would seem that the SBE measures only academic and problem-solving ability on a multiple-choice, paper-and-pencil test, and does not measure effectively the most important area of all, i.e. the student's ability to apply what she knows in actual nursing practice. It would seem desirable to re-examine the underlying philosophy of the SBE, and determine whether in fact it still serves a useful purpose.

Nursing is one of the few helping professions that currently require a culminating examination developed outside a school or college to determine the competency of graduates. The other principal ones are law, medicine, and dentistry. Supposedly, the use of a state examination will ensure that all successful graduates will be able to operate at least at a minimum level of competence.

If we look at some of the other helping professions such as counseling, psychology, teaching, social work, and the ministry, we see that the responsibility for determining the competency of the graduates from a particular program rests with the faculty members who developed the program, and prepared and supervised each student who graduated from that program. This principle has worked out well over the years, and has not resulted in any loss of confidence by the consumer. Although it is true that faculty members in the foregoing fields tend to be more highly educated than most nursing instructors, there is no substantive evidence to indicate that the same faith could not justifiably be placed in nursing instructors. We must also take note of the recent criticisms of nationally administered, multiple-choice testing programs in general, such as those contained in the books by Hoffman, Black, and Gross.

Thus, in reviewing the underlying problems of the SBE, it would seem that the profession of nursing would be wise to move in one of two directions. The first alternative would be to return to the original model of placing the responsibility for preparing students and judging their competency on the faculty within each school. This would eliminate the need for and use of State Board examinations. If such a plan were used, the emphasis would be placed on the accreditation of schools of nursing and the upgrading of graduate programs preparing nursing educators to ensure a competent faculty and a sound educational program. The resources of the NLN could be used more fully to provide guidance and support for individual schools of nursing in their efforts to upgrade themselves.

The other alternative would be to greatly revise the current SBE, following the model used in dentistry and medicine. Thus, in addition to the paper-and-pencil tests of knowledge, there would also be a supervised test of clinical practice. The main problem in this approach lies in the difficulty in administering clinical practice tests to the large number of students who graduate each year, and in securing a sufficient number of qualified clinical evaluators to test them. If the SBE is to be continued, however, then efforts must be made to find a way to incorporate demonstrations of clinical competency within the test. Without such an addition, the SBE may continue to meet only partially its stated objective of ensuring safe practice by those who are able to complete the test successfully.

## STUDIES OF THE NURSING STUDENT

In any discussion of standardized tests, attention must be given to the studies of nursing students which are designed to tell us more about the students with whom we work. The primary emphasis in such research is upon the characteristics of nursing students and their implications for educational planning and programming. These studies fall into two groups, one concerned with a wide variety of tests used for the prediction of success in nursing, and the other concerned with the personality characteristics of those students already enrolled in schools of nursing. The former will be discussed in the next chapter. There are several instruments which have received attention in the latter case.

The first of these is the *Personal Orientation Inventory* (POI) developed by Shostrom. Green (1967) conducted a study on the relation between self-actualization as measured by the POI, and success and satisfaction in the sophomore year of a baccalaureate program. She found the nursing student immature in the degree of self-actualization, which was similar to other college samples. Student nurses also had low scores on scales of Time Competence, Existentiality, and Capacity for Intimate Contact, which suggested an element of anxiety that interfered with the effective use of time, flexibility, and warm relationships. Gunter (1969) also used the POI to compare sophomore nursing students with female college freshmen. She found that nursing students scored significantly higher on all scales of the POI than the college freshmen except on the scales relating to Time Competence, Self Actualizing Values, Self Regard, and the Constructive Nature of Man. Her results in general seem to corroborate those of Green.

Another instrument widely used in research is the *Edwards Personal Preference Schedule* (EPPS). Schulz (1965) used the EPPS in comparing faculty desirability rankings of the 15 traits on the schedule with the performance of two groups of students, sophomore and senior, on the EPPS, and found little relationship. As seen by the faculty, the student nurse should score high in Nurturance, Order, Achievement, Affiliation, and Change. She should score low on Succorance, Aggression, Exhibition, and Abasement. Sophomore students had higher Succorance scores than the seniors, lower Introception, higher Heterosexuality, and higher Change. The general picture given by the students was one of high femininity and pliableness.

Bailey and Claus (1969) used the EPPS to compare nursing students with the general sample of college women. Nursing students consistently scored higher in the need patterns of Nurturance, Order, Abasement, and Succorance. Need patterns in Dominance, Change, and Affiliation never appeared. Adams and Klein (1970) summarize the use of the EPPS by pointing up the inconsistent findings that have resulted from over a dozen studies on nursing students over a decade. They also found changes in students within the same school over a two-year period.

Another instrument that has been used for research is the *Strong Vocational Interest Blank* (SVIB). Aldag (1970) compared occupational and nonoccupational interests of male nurses with those of female nurses, college males, and college females. The study concluded with the observation that interests seem to be vocationally related regardless of sex. Also, male nurses appeared to have interest patterns characterized as more feminine than those of college males on the SVIB masculinity-femininity scale. Two other instruments—the *Leary System of Interpersonal Diagrams* and the *Minnesota Multiphasic Personality Inventory*—were used in a study by Seegars et al. (1963). At the end of the freshman year in a baccalaureate program, the faculty were asked to rate the students academically and clinically, and to differentiate between the managerial-oriented and patient-oriented students. Top students were warmer, more friendly, and more conventional. These students saw their parents as warmer and more loving than the poorer students. Students in the lower group had more autocratic fathers. Patient-oriented nurses were more dominant and independent than the managerial-oriented nurses.

One final semistandardized instrument should be mentioned here, although it is different from the others previously reported. This is the *Flanagan Clinical Experience Record for Nursing Students*. Published in 1960, it was reported on by Flanagan et al. in 1963. The Record was developed as a standardized critical incident record for faculty members in the clinical area. Widely used for some time, it is rapidly being abandoned by many schools. Its use depends on perfect agreement between those behaviors considered important by faculty members using the scale and the emphases on the scale itself. Faculty members have felt a clerical burden in maintaining the scale, find it unsuitable for the average student, and find themselves wasting time trying to determine which category to use for a comment. At best it may provide some help for a faculty interested in developing its own clinical evaluation tools. As a general rule, no standardized instrument such as this should be used within a school of nursing, for, as discussed in Chapter 10, any evaluative tool in the clinical area should be developed by the people who will use it, i.e. the faculty within each school.

## TESTS FOR GUIDANCE

Up to this point we have been discussing the use of standardized tests by faculty members primarily to learn more about their students. One large area that has received minimal attention is the use of tests for guidance purposes, i.e. to help students learn more about themselves, their abilities, and areas in which they may need assistance. There are four tests which may have promise in nursing education. The first of these is the *Brown-Holtzman Survey of Study Habits* (SSH). As many nursing educators recognize, one of the principal difficulties students have is knowing how to study effectively. The SSH can be administered to incoming students quickly (20 to 30 minutes) and easily. Although the test will provide an overall score, the best method would be to concentrate on the special counseling key for the SSH. This is designed to point out the particular trouble spots for individual students. Students can then be provided individual or group assistance in developing sound study habits, or it can be a formal part of the school of nursing orientation program.

A second test that shows promise is the *Cooperative English Test of Reading Comprehension.* This is a 40-minute test that provides percentile band scores in vocabulary, speed of reading, level of comprehension, and total. We know that many of our students also have difficulty in reading skills. This test is most useful as an initial screening device to help identify students with poor reading skills. Identification is meaningless, however, unless the school provides developmental and remedial reading services to its students. This test may not be needed if the student has recently taken a reading test. Note that the SAT, ACT, and the NLN PNG do not do adequate jobs of measuring reading deficiencies.

A third test is the already mentioned *Edwards Personal Preference Schedule.* Based on Murray's need theory, the EPPS provides 15 scores and percentile norms for college men and college women. Standardized on a normal population, the EPPS is most useful in giving students a deeper understanding of themselves, and has served as an excellent introduction to group and individual guidance and counseling.

A fourth test is the *Rotter Incomplete Sentence Blank* (ISB). This should be used solely on an individual basis as an adjunct to counseling. It can provide a valuable tool to the counselor, and an aid to the student in helping her explore areas of difficulty.

The Brown-Holtzman, EPPS, and Rotter ISB are published by the Psychological Corporation of New York, and the Cooperative English Test is published by the Educational Testing Service of Princeton, N.J. These tests, or similar ones, should be used with caution. No test such as these should be used without careful consideration by the faculty and a thorough explanation for the students. Students should always be told exactly why the tests are given, and how the results will be used. If the tests are not followed up by appropriate action, such as remedial work or counseling, then it is usually pointless to use them. They should never be used as a basis for admission or retention of students, for they are primarily useful as guides only. Any test used should be constantly reviewed to determine whether it is still serving the purpose for which it was intended.

## OVERVIEW OF STANDARDIZED TESTS

Certain conclusions can be drawn from the discussion of standardized tests in this chapter. First, there is a paucity of research on the use and effects of standardized testing in nursing education. As a result, many testing programs are based on opinion and subjective judgment. Second, each test needs to be constantly studied as to its usefulness within a particular school of nursing. The fact that other schools may be using a particular test is irrelevant. Third, local norms should be developed for each test in order for the faculty to gain some valid comparison between present and previous students. This is done by some schools now, but should be done by all. Fourth, if any test is given, students should be given a thorough explanation of the test results. Fifth, testing tends to be overdone in many schools. Tests such as the NLN Achievement Tests should be used solely for guidance purposes in helping students spot deficiencies in preparing for State Boards. Sixth, State Board examinations ideally should be eliminated and the final responsibility for determining the competency of a student placed on the qualified faculty within the school that prepared her. Seventh, personality inventories should be used with great caution, and only if there is someone on the faculty, or available as a consultant, who is trained in their use and interpretation.

In summary, standardized tests can be useful tools in the educational process. Nevertheless nursing educators may occasionally lose sight of the inherent limitations in any standardized test, and need to review carefully the use of such tests. When utilized properly, they can be a valuable asset to students and faculty.

# Chapter 12

# *Admissions and Records*

Finding sound methods of choosing the most promising candidates for admission to schools of nursing continues to be problematical for nursing educators. Although the process of selecting students varies from school to school, each one has established certain admission criteria as a basis for selecting suitable applicants. Valid admission criteria are considered essential in relation to the student attrition rate. Supposedly, the attrition rate should be inversely proportionate to the accuracy of selection methods used for admission; i.e. the more accurate the selection methods, the lower the attrition rate. With a current shortage of nurses and an ever-increasing demand for nursing service, it is costly to the student, the school, and the profession to have a high attrition rate.

Dorffeld et al. (1958) found that the failure rate of student nurses on a national level was 33 per cent. Nursing educators seem to agree that better selection procedures may very well reduce the rate of dropouts and permit better use of educational facilities. For this reason, schools of nursing are concerned with setting up admission criteria that will eliminate those candidates who are bound to fail, and yet make the cut-off-point flexible enough to include those students who can succeed if given the opportunity.

## ADMISSION CRITERIA

In general, admission criteria for schools of nursing are based on qualifications in the following five areas:

1. Academic achievement
2. General ability
3. Personality and interests
4. Health
5. Recommendations.

Generally, the faculty of the school of nursing determines the admission criteria for the school. If the school of nursing is located within a college or university, admission criteria will generally coincide with the general admission policy of the institution. For example, in baccalaureate programs the first one or two collegiate years are based on admission criteria determined by the general admissions board of the college or university. After the initial one or two years the student must then meet the admission criteria of the school of nursing. At that point, students fill out applications for admission to the school and are informed about the other procedures for admission.

The selection process is more difficult in those colleges with an open-door policy. Derian (1962) found that 84 per cent of the attrition rate occurred during the first year in a study of associate degree programs in nursing. When nursing programs have an open-door policy, much more needs to be done in the use of individual and group guidance and counseling, especially during the students' first year. It is the responsibility of the faculty to identify those students who are disinterested or unable to succeed and to counsel them out of nursing into other fields for which they may be more suited.

## Personal Characteristics

Requirements relating to age, race, sex, and marital status have changed considerably over the years. Various age limits were set up in the past by individual schools, but generally discrimination on the basis of age is rapidly disappearing. Rejection of students because of their race is also disappearing, partly as a result of civil rights legislation. Barriers against male students are being removed, and the remaining obstacles for married students have been minimized or eliminated. There is no available evidence at present to indicate that these four variables have any validity when used as a basis for selecting students. Therefore there seems to be little value in retaining them as factors affecting admission.

## Academic Achievement

Cognitive factors play the most important single part in the selection criteria for student nurses. This is understandable in view of the findings of Derian that 84 per cent of the students in AD programs left the first year, mostly because of academic failure. Langheim (1966) studied poor achievement in hospital schools of nursing. He found that cognitive factors were still the most decisive in predicting the success of students.

The high school record of achievement still ranks high as a predictor of success in most schools of nursing and is an important part of the admission criteria. In addition to high school grade point average, class ranking is also important in determining the academic achievement of a student. Where she ranked in her graduating class may be more significant than her grade point average. Some schools expect students to rank in the upper half to upper third of their high school class.

Prenursing examinations such as the NLN Pre-Nursing and Guidance Examination discussed in Chapter 11 are also used by some schools as part of the selection criteria. Students are expected to perform at a certain level on such a standardized test in order to be admitted. The other two most commonly used standardized tests used for admission are the American College Test (ACT) and the Scholastic Aptitude Test (SAT) of the College Entrance Examination Boards.

## Required Courses

The student may be required to complete certain courses in high school or college before she is allowed to enter the nursing program. It may, for example, be necessary for the student to have a basic background in the sciences, including behavioral sciences. This is particularly true in many collegiate schools of nursing. Certain levels of science requirements must be met before the student can be admitted. In three-year and AD programs, students may begin taking required science courses such as chemistry and biology concurrently with their nursing courses. In an alternate model they may spend the first year concentrating on science courses while they take a lighter load in the formal nursing courses.

## Personality and Vocational Interests

This particular aspect of admission criteria is somewhat more intangible than the others, and its use varies greatly from school to school. Some schools of nursing administer personality and vocational interest tests routinely. The value and reliability of personality and interest tests in predicting student nurse success are highly questionable, however. Personality data are also usually secured through a preadmission interview and the students' application. Generally, students present references from resource people such as counselors, teachers, and the like, who will vouch for their character. The student herself may be asked to write on topics such as "Why I chose nursing" or "What I want to do ten years from now." Unless such data present evidence of gross emotional immaturity, they are seldom enough in themselves to deter or prevent a student's admission to the school of nursing. Nevertheless this information can be invaluable later on in guidance and counseling provided throughout the students' program.

## Health Requirements

A general medical and dental examination is required of all nursing students prior to admission to most schools of nursing. It is essential that schools have considerable information about a student's physical condition in order to be able to judge whether she will be able to meet some of the strenuous physical requirements of clinical nursing. Faculty members in schools of nursing are well aware that poor physical and emotional health can impair a student's participation in and adjustment to the program. Students often need guidance and counseling about health problems. A good overall health record would seem to be a desirable admission criterion.

## Recommendations

Usually, recommendations from persons who have known the applicant are required as a part of the admission procedure. These are sometimes heavily relied on, since the recommenders not only vouch for the student's character, but usually also predict her chances of success in nursing. The applicant usually selects persons who have known her over a period of time, with whom she has worked as a student or with whom she has had a close relationship. Ministers, teachers, and friends of the family are usually chosen to write recommendations.

Such recommendations should always be taken with caution, however. When students select the persons to write recommendations, they invariably select those who they are reasonably sure will give them a positive recommendation. It would seem desirable for the school of nursing to specify partially or completely the persons from whom recommendations should be solicited, such as the school counselor, principal, family physician, employer, and the like. This will produce more valid and reliable recommendations.

## Preadmission Interview

An essential part of establishing whether or not a student meets the admission requirements is the use of the preadmission interview. During the interview, assessments of the student's personality, interests, motivation, and emotional maturity can be made. The interview presents an opportunity for the interviewer and student to discuss the student's concept of nursing. The interview can also be used to evaluate the applicant's potential for nursing.

Generally, as Kaback (1958) points out, the faculty of the school determines the objectives of the preadmission interview and decides upon the kind of questions to be raised with the applicant. It is important for the interviewer to be skilled in the techniques of interviewing. The interview may be done by a counselor in the school of nursing or a faculty member trained in interviewing procedures. Sometimes both a counselor and an instructor, functioning as a team, can handle the screening and interviewing of applicants. The importance of the interview should never be underestimated. Meadow and Goss (1971) report on the problems of the novice interviewer, and believe that persons responsible for conducting interviews can be assisted in improving their methods by others prepared in this area.

When data on the prospective student are complete, then comes the task of whether or not to accept the student. This may be a difficult decision, because, in spite of all the data gathered, there still remains the element of rationally weighing all available criteria. The student may meet all the admission criteria except that she scored low on the PNG or SAT. Then the faculty has to determine whether or not to give the student a chance in spite of the low test score. Some schools of nursing have an admissions committee which is charged with the responsibility of determining the final acceptance or rejection of an applicant based upon established admission criteria. Admissions are seldom cut and dried, and should not be, and the admission committee is often the final decision maker. The composition of the admission committee should represent a cross section of the school's faculty; e.g. it may include the admissions counselor and three faculty members, the latter ideally selected by the faculty to represent them. In addition, faculty members should rotate on the committee so that all will eventually have the opportunity to participate in evaluating students for admission.

One precautionary note that should be mentioned here is that admission committees would be wise to eliminate the use of any rigid cut-off scores as criteria for admission. Seldom, if ever, can such scores be defended, especially with the lack of precision in any of our current criteria. Committees would operate on a much sounder basis if they reviewed all available criteria as openly as possible, and made professional judgments without relying on rigid scores to determine admission or rejection. The rigid use of such scores is highly impersonal, and denies the human element that, in the final analysis, could determine the success or failure of the student.

## RECRUITMENT

Knowles (1961) says that it is difficult to find a valid method of predicting how many professional persons society will need from time to time. For example, various sociological events such as depression, war or disease epidemics influence the number of nurses needed. It is well known that in some parts of the country there is an overwhelming scarcity of nurses. Heidgerken (1969) reported that there is a smaller percentage of women entering the nursing profession despite the fact that there are more women working today than ever before. More research is clearly needed in looking at factors that are important in choosing nursing as a career, especially longitudinal studies which include job satisfaction. The perception of professional roles is an important factor in career decisions, and students should have an understanding of the nature of nursing and its various programs.

### Who Is Responsible for Recruitment?

Some schools of nursing employ a counselor specifically for recruitment. In larger schools the recruitment of students constitutes a full-time job, especially if the recruitment extends over a wide geographical area. The recruiter may spend much time traveling to various high schools, future nurse clubs, and so forth, interpreting the school of nursing program. An important function of the recruiter is to help students understand admission criteria and inform them of the availability of financial aid. Although the recruiter does not have to be a nurse, she should be familiar with the school of nursing program.

Part of the task of recruitment is to upgrade nursing and make it appealing to high school students. Coulter (1966) says that recent events related to campus demonstrations, participation in the Peace Corps and Vista, and freedom marches indicate that the recruitment of high school students for nursing should focus on presenting nursing as a profession for those who wish to help other human beings. Coulter believes that placing the stress on service to humanity will help to recruit today's students. Concern for others can be a strong motivating force in nursing that can be utilized in recruitment efforts.

The recruiter has the responsibility of interpreting nursing to the students and making it attractive, not only by emphasizing the positive aspects, but also by clearly explaining the different levels of nursing and differences in programs. High school students need to be thoroughly oriented to the opportunities provided by the different kinds of nursing programs. Their ultimate choice will depend on the recruitment efforts by the profession, their understanding of the role and function of the nurse, and the understanding of the programs by parents, teachers, and high school counselors.

Unfortunately, many high school and college counselors are confused about the different levels of nursing. They need to understand the inherent differences between the three main nursing programs, e.g. diploma, AD, and baccalaureate. They need to understand clearly the admission criteria for each program. If students are interested in later transferring into higher degree programs, they need to know what is involved, e.g. how much credit they can receive, and the opportunity to take proficiency or challenge examinations. This is information that is necessary for long-term planning.

### Recruitment Methods

The recruiter and the counselor also need a clear conceptual image of the student nurse. Klemer (1964) found in a small study that guidance counselors did not have a distorted conceptual image of the basic nursing student. On the other hand, some of the opinions of nurse educators lacked agreement, which suggests that faculty members should examine their own agreement on the conceptual image of the student nurse before attempting to influence high school and college counselors. In another study by C. J. Peterson (1969), assessing the knowledge of trends in nursing education by college counselors and nurse educators, counselors relied on written career information more than on direct contact with nurses and nursing educators. Both groups believed that opportunities for humanitarian expression and the desire to work with people were important factors in attracting students into nursing.

Guidance personnel in high schools need to be well informed about all aspects of nursing programs in order to provide their students with meaningful and correct information. Leonetti (1965) reported that most high school guidance departments lacked the information which future nursing students need and request. This is an aspect of recruitment that can and must be improved. It is the responsibility of the nursing profession to share necessary information with high school counselors. Kennedy (1961) described a method of using workshops for guidance counselors and high school teachers. The workshops proved helpful in disseminating information about the nursing profession. The counselors were better able to understand the various educational opportunities available in nursing. The kind of program selected by a student is of critical importance to her career.

Parker (1964) reports recruitment efforts through high school "College Days." Meeting students individually and in groups provided an opportunity to increase their understanding of the school of nursing. In addition, time was provided for discussions with guidance counselors and teachers. Klassen and White (1971) described a "Health Day" in Dodge City, Missouri. With booths representing the various health careers, each kind of nursing program was presented. Films were also used to increase effectiveness. The use of future nurse clubs is an additional avenue for the recruitment of high school students which is both popular and effective.

An article by Fillmore (1963) contains information about career publications which are available from the NLN, state nursing committees, and schools of nursing, and which counselors can use as a source of accurate and current information. Vickery (1970) writes about an exploratory work experience program at Alhambra High School in Martinez, California. Of the 63 students who have participated to date, 23 have entered nursing schools or have chosen other health careers. The students are able to gain a more realistic picture of nursing through actual experience. The students assist nurses as members of a team. They observe selected procedures, run errands, and spend a day with the student nurses at the University of California School of Nursing. In some respects this is similar to orientation programs in which students get to spend some time touring and discussing nursing prior to actual entrance into a school of nursing. These students seem better prepared to adjust to the hospital setting. Posters, newspaper articles, speakers, radio, television, and so on, are all media used by nursing schools for recruitment.

Special recruitment efforts are being directed toward getting male students, older students, married students, and those students from disadvantaged groups to apply to schools of nursing. Richter (1969) reports recruitment offers to reach and attract mature women by means of posters, television, radio, and newspaper feature articles. The program resulted in responses from women aged 20 to 61. Meadow and Edelson (1963) found that age and marital status appeared to be important factors in the prediction of academic success in nursing. It needs to be emphasized that careers in nursing are available for mature persons who are interested in the nursing profession.

The recruitment of disadvantaged students creates more of a challenge for recruiters. Minority groups have not been represented in nursing in proportion to their numbers in the general population. With the current shortage of nurses, educators have begun to look for potential students not only among males and older women, but also among minority and disadvantaged groups.

Yates (1970) reports that 0.5 per cent of nursing students in Minnesota represented minority groups when the Civil Rights Act of 1964 passed, whereas 7 per cent of the students involved in public schools were Negro, Indian, and Spanish. What does this indicate? Nursing faculties were understanding about the low percentage of minority students, but were somewhat reluctant to offer them an opportunity for careers in nursing.

Educators were concerned about the standards of nursing education and believed that the minority student would jeopardize them. Subsequently, Minnesota nursing students started "Project Motivation," in which they tried various measures for recruitment that proved to have little effect on minority students.

The sort of recruitment used for the disadvantaged student has to differ from the usual approach. It would indeed be futile to rely on visual aids that picture the typical student nurse as a white, middle-class student. This is the portrayal usually seen in recruiting films. Recruiters need to be more realistic in spelling out admission criteria and job opportunities. The disadvantaged group may be more apt to respond to action-oriented recruitment programs in which the recruiter brings along some nursing equipment as visual aids. This stimulates interest because the students are able to pick up and handle the equipment, such as blood pressure apparatus, thermometer or stethoscope. A non-nurse may be able to handle this sort of recruitment effectively, or a counselor may want to have a nurse participate in a demonstration program. The recruiter helps create in the potential student's mind a better image of nursing, one more realistic than some of the childhood fantasies about the glamour of nursing.

At the 1965 NLN convention, Johnson (1966) reported that the NSNA adopted a resolution that the group begin a project to assist young people from minority groups to prepare themselves for a career in nursing. These students have provided high school counselors with information and helped place information about nursing in black newspapers and on radio stations. The student nurses have been active in recruiting blacks for schools of nursing.

Earlier in this chapter it was mentioned that nursing educators were somewhat reluctant to open doors for minority group students because of the fear that their admission would lower the standards of the school. A large number of the minority student applicants seem not to pass all the current admission criteria, particularly in the area of academic achievement. Because of the inequality of the school systems of minority students, perhaps other methods of selection should be instituted.

Because the validity and fairness of selection tests have been questioned when used with different ethnic groups, New York University, between 1965 and 1967, concluded a study of two black schools and two white schools with the NLN PNG. The correlation between the two white schools of nursing indicated that the PNG was generally valid as a predictor of success. White students scored higher on all parts of the PNG than the black students, but they did not score higher on all parts of the State Board licensure examination. The race of the applicant should thus be considered when reviewing PNG examination scores, and nursing education programs should be geared to overcome the deficiencies of these students.

Nursing schools can establish remedial programs if they are sincere about helping the minority student. A tutorial and remedial program should be implemented by those schools that want to extend opportunities in nursing to minority groups. The tutorial and remedial programs could be part of the overall recruitment process. Henke (1971) reports that St. Vincent's Hospital School of Nursing in New York City offered a tutorial advancement program which consisted of an eight-week remedial program during the summer and a tutorial assistance program the first year. The summer program included grammar, reading comprehension, computation skills, and study skills. Field trips, outings, and group discussions were arranged. Six of the nine students who participated in the program were subsequently admitted to the school of nursing. Defrank (1971) also reports on arrangements made at St. Francis Hospital School of Nursing in Delaware. Remedial instruction in reading and mathematics was offered those applicants whose reading comprehension scores were below the twentieth percentile. Thirteen of the 20 participants were subsequently accepted into the school of nursing.

Harvey (1970) says that new and massive remedial projects are needed and that a wide-open admission door should be operating. She advocates help with problem-solving and critical thinking skills both before and after enrollment, accompanied by help with written skills. Once the disadvantaged students have acquired these abilities, they will have a much greater feeling of belonging to the class. Some educators may perhaps believe that remedial programs require too great an investment of time and effort. Yet if there is a shortage of nurses and if remedial programs help decrease the attrition rate, then the programs are worthwhile and should be supported by faculties. Faculty members must take the initiative in making special arrangements to assist the disadvantaged student in order to provide equal educational opportunities for all.

ODWIN is a program described by Osgood (1969) in which a remedial program to aid minority group students was supplemented by individual and group counseling and behavioral conditioning therapy. Guidance and counseling are extremely important parts of any program that attempts to help students from disadvantaged groups cope with their feelings of inferiority or of being in the minority. Feelings of rejection and overprotection are common, and there is a need to express these feelings and learn to overcome them.

Remedial programs are necessary for the disadvantaged student, but both remedial and diagnostic programs should be developed for all students who seem to be having academic difficulty. Again, guidance and counseling should be provided in conjunction with the remedial program so that students can learn to cope with their feelings. As discussed in Chapter 11, diagnostic tests in basic skills are important for students who are having academic difficulties. A group of students having similar difficulties may profit from group guidance and group support. Students are able to meet to look at their areas of difficulty. Remedial work can be useful in removing one threat by assisting students to complete their academic work successfully. For example, as a result of a remedial group in psychiatric nursing, all the participating students passed the course successfully during the year in one school of nursing. Some schools of nursing set up remedial programs for students based on their NLN PNG or NLN Achievement test performance; i.e. if the students fall below a certain percentile, they are placed in a remedial program. Although the main aim was to assist students to pass State Boards, some diploma schools have set up remedial groups and have achieved good results. Remedial groups can be beneficial if they are viewed as an exploratory method of dealing with problems and not as a punitive measure. The emphasis needs to be placed on the feelings and problems of learning rather than the end-goal of getting through the nursing program.

Proficiency tests should also be provided for those students who are exceptional and are able to study and challenge a course. This prevents a student from having to sit through a course that she has already mastered. Some schools of nursing offer proficiency examinations for both theory and clinical practice. Students may also get credit for parts of the examination. Usually the student is denied the opportunity to challenge the clinical examination if she cannot successfully challenge the theory part. Here again, guidance and counseling are essential in helping the exceptional student to grow and develop fully.

## STUDENT RECORDS

The student record is kept for the benefit of the student. Information placed in the student's record is kept in confidence among the faculty, and information may be added to the record in order to assist the student in the program. The record usually contains a record of the student's admission criteria such as test results, high school grades, high school rank in class, health records, letters of recommendation, student letters and communications, college record, requirements completed, official actions taken, and so forth.

During the student's program the record is continually kept up to date. Evaluations from various courses and clinical evaluations are added to the record. Notes from advisors regarding registration or student problems are also kept in the record. Some schools of nursing encourage the advisors to keep a complete record, including detailed notes of student and faculty concerns. The record should include anything that might be significant in helping the student adjust to and proceed through the program. At the end of the nursing program all these notes should be destroyed and a final summary prepared for the permanent record. In this way, instructors and advisors feel freer to add material to the student's record that they feel is essential in helping others understand her or add to her progress and adjustment.

The final summary includes only that information pertinent to the student's performance. For example, if a student had difficulty with writing skills, but was able to master the problem, then this information becomes irrelevant and it would be unnecessary to add the information to the final summary. The information would be helpful only to those instructors who were concerned with having the student master writing skills.

There is a question of who writes the final summary. The person responsible will vary in different schools of nursing. Usually it is the responsibility of the director of the school or her delegated representative such as the student's advisor. Summarizing the student record is an extremely important task and is highly significant for the student, since this record will follow her throughout life. Faculty should take this re-

sponsibility seriously and decide who is best qualified to fulfill the responsibility.

## STUDENT RECOMMENDATIONS

Who makes student recommendations, and what is their purpose?
Student recommendations are highly regarded as an important part of
the admission criteria for schools of higher education. They are also highly valued by future employers. Now that pass-fail systems are beginning
to be used by schools of nursing, written student recommendations have
achieved particular importance. In some schools both instructors and
advisors are encouraged to make student recommendations throughout
the student's program. This is particularly true if the instructor or advisor
feels that the student would be wise to seek advanced study in nursing,
or if they feel that negative recommendations are indicated. Questions
always arise in this area. Does the person doing the summary of the student's record restrict her recommendations solely to the data presented?
Are students made aware of the recommendations, particularly if they
are negative? Faculty members must give serious thought to these
questions and honestly and carefully consider their impact throughout
a student's future career.

Perhaps some help can be found in the excellent study by Brown
(1961). He makes eight recommendations that deal directly with problems
of student records and recommendations. They provide an excellent
synthesis of our discussion.

1. Colleges and universities should critically review their student record system as it relates to dealing with inquiries.

2. Distinctions need to be made between the public and private
aspects of the student record.

3. Interpreting, rather than reporting information, is essential to
good practice.

4. Each inquiry should be evaluated in terms of its relevancy to
available information about the student.

5. Specific information about the purposes of the inquiry and possible uses of information released are essential to good practice.

6. Students should be involved in policies and practices with respect
to the external use of information and the formulation of policy for dealing with inquiries.

7. Institutional policy is preferable to personal judgment as a basis
for practice.

8. Policies and practices for interpreting the student have important
implications for the student-college relationship.

# Chapter 13

# Attrition in
# Schools of Nursing

In the previous chapter the increasing need for nurses, based on the needs of an increasing population, was referred to as a priority concern of nursing schools. The goal of nursing educators is to increase recruitment, enrollment, and retention of nursing students, and at the same time to reduce the number of students who are unsuccessful in nursing programs. Faculties are concerned not only about improving their recruitment and educational programs, but also about reducing the number of dropouts through a better selection process and better student service programs. Because of the interest created by the high attrition rates in schools of nursing, educators have been prompted to re-examine the admission process and to increase the research conducted in this area. Current methods of selection have been criticized, and schools of nursing are being challenged to find the most effective methods for the selection of promising nursing students.

## ATTRITION STUDIES

In a survey conducted throughout the country, Klahn (1969) reported that more than one third of entering nursing students drop out of nursing prior to completion of their program. Dorffeld (1958) reported an attrition rate of 33 per cent. If our aim is to increase the supply of nurses, then it is obvious that attrition rates require serious study in an attempt to identify contributing factors that seem to cause student failure. For example, students leave nursing programs because of unsatisfactory performance in the classroom and clinical area or because of some personal or emotional concern. Thurston et al. (1962) discuss the withdrawal problem in schools of nursing, citing lack of motivation and personality problems as contributing factors. The authors also point up the problem of studying withdrawal in light of individual differences between schools as well as between students.

Lindstrom (1961), in a dissertation, examined student survival in collegiate nursing programs to determine reasons for withdrawal and differences between those who stay and those who leave. Variables studied included age, performance, HSGPA, college GPA, reason for going to college, reactions to college, need for self-support, and amount of extracurricular activity in which the student participates. Lindstrom found that reasons for withdrawal were usually multiple, and both groups were dissatisfied with academic counseling. This is an important finding, and indicates clearly the need for schools of nursing to re-examine their advising and counseling programs.

Hill, Taylor, and Stacy (1963) at the Universities of Utah and California conducted a large-scale research project concerning attrition in schools of nursing as well as job turnover in professional nursing. The massive project included the study of over 300 published and unpublished studies, and reports on methods of selection and guidance of nursing students, measures of academic ability, and successful clinical nursing performance. The reasons for withdrawal ranked in order of their performance are failure in classwork, marriage, dislike of nursing, ill health, unsuitable personality, disappointment in nursing, failure in practical work, violation of rules, transfer to or preference for another school or field, homesickness, family responsibility, personal reasons, financial reasons, and immaturity.

Although further short-range and longitudinal studies are needed, a number of the reasons listed are directly related to personality characteristics. At present, personality characteristics have not been sufficiently defined to be used for the prediction of success among students prior to their actual enrollment. Nevertheless study and review of the literature seem to support the need for a well-functioning guidance and counseling program in order to help students adjust and remain in school.

Katzell (1967) found that satisfactions rather than stresses affect the attrition rates in schools of nursing. As director of the National League for Nursing Evaluation Service, Katzell conducted a study of 1852 students in 43 diploma programs. During the students' first week they completed a questionnaire concerning the stresses and satisfactions they expected during the first year; later they were asked to respond to the same items in relation to what they had actually experienced. She found that students reported both less stress and less satisfaction received during the program. Again, these findings seem to indicate the need for program revision in schools of nursing.

Rottkamp (1969) discussed reasons for high attrition rates in baccalaureate programs in which academic failure accounted for 35 to 38 per cent of the student dropouts. A wide range of academic ability was revealed in state board examination scores. Insufficient academic challenge was given as one of the key reasons for attrition, although Rottkamp found that there was usually more than one cause for student withdrawal. Again, a study such as this points up the need for preventing disillusionment for the beginning student. Research into more effective selection procedures might lead to the elimination of those students most prone to disillusionment. The study seems to indicate the need for more accurate recruitment and orientation programs, more complete guidance and counseling services, and a more creative and exciting academic program as the best means of significantly reducing student loss of interest and satisfaction.

## PREDICTING SUCCESS IN NURSING PROGRAMS

Success of a student in nursing is usually defined either in terms of passing the state board licensure examination or achieving satisfactory grades throughout her nursing program. In the previous chapter on admission criteria, it was stated that ideally the more accurate the selection process, the lower should be the rate of attrition. Despite the ambiguity of the term "success," educators have continued to search for selection methods that would help to predict the success or failure of a student in nursing programs.

Standardized preadmission tests have been relied on as a tool for predicting a student's chance to succeed in nursing. If standardized tests alone could be used for predicting success, then the problem of establishing admission critera would either be greatly minimized or would no longer exist. Nursing educators disagree, however, as to the total value of standardized preadmission tests. We know that the greatest student attrition occurs during the first year, usually as a result of academic failure. There is some question and a good deal of confusion about the validity and reliability of such tests. Although the tests seem able to separate academically high achievers from low achievers, no test seems able to predict satisfactorily the success or failure of an individual student. Other parameters that enter in include attitude, motivation, and interest. Some educators believe that the HSGPA is just as reliable as the standardized tests as a predictor of success.

### Prenursing and Guidance Examination

The staff of the NLN Measurement and Evaluation Service (1970) examined the validity of the NLN prenursing and guidance examination in relation to students' classroom and clinical performance. The students in the study were in the top, middle, and lower thirds of the class. A rating was obtained for five different periods during the students' enrollment and compared with the mean scores on each of the tests of the PNG examination. PNG scores of the students in the top third were significantly higher than those in the bottom third. This was also true in ratings of clinical performance. The staff also examined PNG performance in relation to overall performance in a school of nursing, and found that PNG examination scores show a relationship with academic failure, but not with withdrawals for nonacademic reasons.

A study by Muhlenkamp (1967) at St. Mary's Hospital School of Nursing in Milwaukee related to academic failure. The use of multiple cutoffs on the PNG was examined. A cutoff score is established for each part of the examination which the candidate must exceed. Perhaps the use of multiple cutoffs will reduce attrition caused by academic failure. Research on students is needed over a period of years to determine the validity of the cutoff scores. Perhaps a better indication can be reached by weighting the various scores or by developing a multiple regression equation. In any event, a student's test profile can still be useful in indicating an area of weakness which would be important in planning counseling or remedial work.

In 1967 Grundeman and the staff of the NLN Test Services reviewed the use of the PNG in the prediction of attrition in diploma programs. A study was conducted of students admitted to Madison General Hospital School of Nursing in Wisconsin from 1960 to 1962 to assess the value of PNG examination scores and high school rank converted to percentiles. It was found that the PNG composite raw score, academic aptitude, quantitative scaled score, mathematics raw score and natural science scaled score all appeared to be valuable predictors of success. Although tests were found to be useful in predicting a student's potential to graduate, they were unable to predict which students will in fact graduate.

DeLourdes and Ary (1967) examined the PNG in relation to high school rank and licensure examination performance. A study was conducted at St. Frances Hospital School of Nursing, La Crosse, Wisconsin. The results of 114 students who took the licensure examination from 1963 to 1965 suggest that high school rank alone would have been a useful predictor, but PNG results would have been a better one. In another report by the staff of the NLN Test Services (1970), three generalizations about the PNG were supported.

1. PNG scores of entrants into schools of nursing exceeded those of applicants.

2. At each stage of the program, PNG scores of those students who were academically successful exceeded those of students who withdrew because of academic failure.

3. PNG scores of those who withdrew for nonacademic reasons did not differ significantly from those who remained in nursing.

In view of these studies it would seem that the PNG cannot be used to predict nonacademic failures or withdrawals. At best it may be useful for group prediction of successful completion of students in diploma programs; other selection criteria are needed for individual prediction. Current research does not support the concept of using the PNG as a rigid selection tool, nor does the NLN recommend its use for this purpose. In Chapter 11 we described the relations between the PNG, NLN Achievement Tests, and the State Board examination. Much more research is needed to support clearly any relationship between the PNG and success either as a nursing student or as a graduate nurse. We particularly need some agreement on a satisfactory criterion of success.

## SAT–ACT–GPA

Munday and Hoyt (1965) found that nursing schools differ widely in terms of their students' academic potential. Regardless of this difference, students score lower in the mathematical area than in other areas of academic ability. They found that the ACT was an excellent predictor of overall grades in the student's first year of nursing. At the University of Virginia School of Nursing, records of 219 students graduating between 1962 and 1966 were used in a study to determine whether College

Board examination scores and high school averages would provide useful and significant information related to the prediction of achievement in nursing. The SAT was found to be more predictive of state board scores, and high school GPA more predictive of school of nursing GPA.

Kovacs (1968) investigated the use of measures of intelligence, rank in high school class, and performance on the SAT among students in baccalaureate programs. Once again, the SAT correlated with scores on the State Board examination and was a better predictor of achievement than high school rank. Goza (1970) found that students who passed State Board examinations had higher ACT scores and NLN Achievement scores. He noted that NLN test scores seem to be related to success on the SBE, and that academically superior student nurses had greater success on the SBE. In a study of prediction of success in a collegiate program of nursing, Burgess and Duffey (1969) found that the pre-nursing GPA was the single most significant predictor of nursing GPA.

Other studies have indicated that the HSGPA is just as valid a predictor of academic success in nursing as other selection devices. Michael et al. (1965) found that the HSGPA in "solid subjects" was the most valid indicator of success in academic and clinical performance in nursing on trying to summarize the reported research relating to the SAT, ACT, and GPA as predictors of success. There seems to be considerable disagreement as to the value of any one of the three as a valid predictor. We have already discussed in the previous chapter the interrelations of the ACT, SAT, PNG, NLN Achievement Tests, and SBE. Even though there may be reasonable correlations among these tests, the question still remains unanswered as to their ability to predict success. We again return to the lack of longitudinal data and agreed criteria of success.

## PERSONALITY, ATTITUDE, AND INTEREST TESTS AS PREDICTORS OF SUCCESS

Many students leave nursing for reasons other than academic failure. Some express dissatisfaction and disappointment in nursing and seem to be confused both about the role of nursing and why they chose nursing as a career. Educators have attempted to find a means of determining student motivation through an examination of their personality and interests. Personality tests became a means of selecting applicants in the hope of reducing the attrition rate that occurs for nonacademic reasons. Is there a certain nursing personality type or a collection of personality traits and interests that could qualify or disqualify a student applicant for entrance into a school of nursing? According to the literature, the use of interest and aptitude tests has not been successful in predicting success in nursing.

Crider (1943) found that the Strong Vocational Interest Blank could not discriminate between successful and unsuccessful nurses. Kirk et al. (1961) used the Strong and the Otis Self Administering Test of Mental Ability and found that neither test predicted withdrawal from the nursing program for academic unsuitability or grade point average. Diverse patterns of interest seem not to be related to the success of students in a nursing program. Lukens (1965) concluded in a study of personality traits that individuals with quite different needs and values appear to be well accommodated within the broad occupational field of nursing. Both the Kuder Preference Record and the Strong Vocational Interest Blank were used by Mowbray and Taylor (1967) without much success in predicting success in schools of nursing. The social service score on the Kuder Preference Record proved to be the only variable related to adjustment in the nursing program. Dorffeld (1958) found that the Kuder Preference Record had no selective value, and the Edwards Personal Preference Schedule showed slight discriminating power which proved not to be significant. Crider (1943) also used the Bell Adjustment Inventory without much success.

Although schools of nursing continue to use vocational interest tests as part of the admission and selection criteria, studies to date have failed to support the validity and reliability of their use for this purpose. Nursing educators have also consistently called for research into the importance of personality factors in nursing. Again, studies to date have failed to prove the effectiveness of personality tests as measures of traits necessary for success in nursing. Even the use of projective techniques has failed to predict successfully students' success in nursing. Although the Rorschach test is impractical for general use, Berg (1947) failed to discriminate between graduates and nongraduates in nursing by using the Rorschach test.

Langheim (1966), in his study of three diploma schools using the Minnesota Multiphasic Personality Inventory (MMPI), found that it could not predict underachievement in preclinical or clinical courses. He stated that when dealing with cognitive achievement, the I.Q. factor was of great importance, and that students with a marginal personality adjustment can still succeed in nursing if they have enough intelligence. He found that at times personality deviation seemed to help students and that some defenses could be an asset. He did find that poor achievement correlated with extreme MMPI scores, but that each of these students could have been easily identified without the use of the MMPI. In the clinical area he also found that the intellective factor was significant, along with the cognitive factor. Only students with extreme scores in hypochondria, depression, and hysteria could be predicted underachievers. It may be desirable, then, not to choose students with borderline intellectual ability if there are also extreme scores on personality tests. Bernfeld (1967) also used the MMPI to predict student nurse performance in a hospital program. His results failed to confirm the hypotheses that dropouts and perseverants could be distinguished by the MMPI.

Klahn (1969) thought that the self-concept might be an important aspect to consider in first-year students, but the self-concept scale and the Change Seeker Index failed to make a precise discrimination between successful and unsuccessful student nurses. Students who stayed in nursing did have a slightly more positive ideal self-concept. Dropouts scored higher in a professed need for greater change. Klahn used the premise that an integrated self-concept and healthy concept of role is a prerequisite for adequate functioning in the nursing role,

Thurston et al. (1965) could find no significant differences in MMPI performance between achievers and underachievers, failures and underachievers, or failures and achievers. Significant achievement group differences were noted in terms of PNG scores and high school rank in class. Girona (1969) looked at the Semantic Differential as a tool in predicting the potential effectiveness of student nurses. The affect scale scores only partially correlated with instructors' evaluations of the subjects' potential effectiveness.

Johnson and Leonard (1970) used a battery of psychological tests (1) to describe the psychological characteristics of those beginning the professional course sequence in a baccalaureate nursing program; (2) to determine the effectiveness of these characteristics in predicting theory and practice grades. The students completed a psychological test battery that included the 16 Personality Factor scale and the Strong Vocational Interest Blank. Test scores indicated that they were average in scholastic aptitude compared with other University of Wisconsin females. Their personality test scores indicated that they were more intelligent, assertive, and experimenting than college women in general. The test scores were of little value in predicting the practice grade. The authors felt that a search for factors associated with clinical practice grades needs to be continued.

In 1961 French investigated the effectiveness of a battery of predictive tests used by a diploma school of nursing. The following tests were used: California Test of Mental Maturity, Terman McNemar Test of Mental Ability, California Achievement Battery, and the Iowa Test of Educational Development. He selected the final GPA and the grade on the State Boards as criteria of success. His conclusion was that this particular battery of tests showed substantial validity with both GPA and State Boards. Some authors believe that the HSGPA is an effective predictor of academic success in nursing, and that, by adding the PNG, a better prediction is possible. There is little if any solid evidence at the present, however, to support the addition of psychological tests as selectors.

## COMBINED PREDICTORS OF SUCCESS IN NURSING

Taylor et al. (1966), in a survey of selection methods used in schools of nursing, collected data on 698 schools of nursing and 180 published reports. Taylor concluded that there is a lack of research showing a clear relation between academic success and on-the-job success in nursing. The most frequently used selection criteria were a battery of tests. Each school seemed to be evaluating its screening needs, and was eliminating unnecessary selection methods to increase efficiency. Garrett (1960) found that the HSGPA, Hunt Arithmetic Test, Iowa Silent Reading Test, and Minnesota Clerical Test were fairly effective in predicting success in one school.

Gerstein (1965) also examined the efficiency of a battery of paper-

and-pencil tests as a selection method for women entering a three-year nursing program. The tests used were the Otis, the IPAT Culture Free Test, Diagnostic Reading Survey, and the Strong Vocational Interest Blank. Only performance in the diagnostic reading test indicated significant differences between dropouts and graduates.

Since most student withdrawals occur because of academic failure, and since the cognitive tests such as the SAT and PNG have some predictive value in this area, then they would most likely be used by schools of nursing. Perhaps the schools need to reconsider how and why they are using a psychological battery of tests. Are they really useful within the particular school, or are they merely given in hopes that longitudinal research studies will eventually find in them some predictive factors? Should these tools be continued until better instruments are found or developed? Are they really essential in screening out students with obvious personality problems? Perhaps the initial interview would have as great or greater validity in identifying gross personality maladjustment.

Taylor (1966) identifies the most frequently used selection criteria in the 698 schools of nursing surveyed. The results as indicated by the schools were as follows:

|  | *Most Important* | *Frequency of Use* |
|---|---|---|
| HSGPA | 49% | 91% |
| Application forms | 23 | 90 |
| Interview | 18 | 92 |
| Health forms | 15 | 88 |
| Biographical inventory | 12 | 59 |
| References | 12 | 88 |
| Test Battery: NLNPNG | 47 | 41 |
| Psych. Corp. | | |
| Others not | | |
| designed for nursing | 48 | 46 |
| Other procedures | 26 | 17 |

According to the survey, the HSGPA was considered to be the most important criterion by schools, and was one of the three most widely used criteria.

Litherland (1966) found that the HSGPA was basically more powerful in predicting success. It alone affords a counselor predictive accuracy at least equal to that of other prediction variables in combination. Thomas (1967), using a single class in a single diploma school, found no significant increase in correlation between HSGPA and class rank in nursing when a psychological battery was added. She found that NLN composite scores and psychological battery ratings added nothing of significance to the HSGPA as a predictor of success in nursing.

It is difficult to predict attrition for individual students by using present selection criteria. Nevertheless educators continue to be concerned with the attrition rate and the loss of academically capable students for academic and nonacademic reasons. It is here that guidance counselors begin to play an important role. Researchers have continued to recommend good guidance and counseling programs for student nurses throughout their programs to help them understand and integrate their nursing roles. The counselor is able to help the student deal with problems as they arise. Diligent research is needed into the effects counseling can have on the attrition rate.

## CONCLUSIONS

It is difficult to find much consensus in the contradictory research reported on attrition. It seems that nursing educators have been concentrating their efforts on finding new, concrete ways of predicting success and failure as the best method of reducing the attrition rate. We would suggest the following as some of the steps that need to be followed in dealing with the problem of attrition.

1. Greater improvement is needed in acquainting student applicants with career opportunities in nursing. Better recruitment and orientation methods will help students gain a better understanding of themselves in relation to the various career opportunities in nursing.

2. The development of a strong guidance and counseling program would be useful in assisting students toward greater self-understanding and achievement of maturity, as well as assisting them in dealing with personal concerns that are affecting their performance.

3. It would seem desirable to eliminate the use of all psychological tests until research supports their use, and to concentrate on the use of one good measure of scholastic aptitude.

4. There is a genuine need for coordinated national research into attrition problems and program solutions.

5. Much greater emphasis is needed on remedial and tutorial programs to help students overcome academic deficiencies that lead to failure.

6. New and creative educational programs need to be developed that will challenge students, maintain their interest, and help them achieve.

7. A decided effort is needed in defining criteria of success in nursing. The use of GPA and State Board results seems too arbitrary, and there is no research clearly showing a significant relation between test results or GPA and long-term success in nursing. Unless we can agree on what constitutes success in nursing or the qualities of a good nurse, we will always have difficulty in satisfactorily predicting success.

Attrition continues to be a large problem for concerned nursing educators. We constantly witness the loss of numbers of talented and motivated young people from our schools of nursing. It is our hope that the foregoing suggestions, and the philosophy and programs described throughout this book will help to reduce the rate of attrition in schools of nursing.

# Chapter 14

## Student Development in Nursing Education

Student personnel policies, practices, and programs are being challenged from every conceivable direction, by students, faculty, and student personnel workers as well as by external forces—parents, public, and legislature. The field of student personnel is in a state of flux, and well it should be! Over the years since the turn of the century, student personnel workers have functioned as *regulators in loco parentis;* as *service personnel,* wherein their role was to provide specialized services geared to higher education institutional expectations or the desires of industrial and governmental institutions as in the case of financial aid and placement bureaus; or as *therapists* with the primary emphasis on dealing with specific personal problems after the fact.

The most influential statement on student personnel principles had been the "Student Personnel Point of View" as proposed by the American Council on Education in 1937 and 1949. These principles viewed the student as an individual who must be regarded as a whole person with not only intellectual needs, but also needs pertaining to his social, emotional, physical, and spiritual development. Unfortunately, the emphasis has been on assisting students by providing a different "service" area to meet each need, i.e., counselor for the emotional, advisor for the social activities, intramural advisors and physical education personnel for the physical, and chaplains for the spiritual, with only the faculty dealing with intellectual needs. Administrators such as the dean of students were responsible for student discipline. Consequently the whole person concept encouraged fragmented attention, and students were treated statistically rather than behaviorally. Students rebelled against such treatment, as did personnel workers against the limitations of such a system of service.

More recently a new concept has been developing, which has wide ramifications for student personnel workers. It is called the Student Development Point of View and is receiving considerable attention. One of the best descriptions of the new model has been offered by writers in the community-junior college field, O'Banion, Thurston, and Gulden, who in early 1970 proposed an emerging model of student personnel in which the worker is called a human development facilitator. Their model supports functions which are facilitative, preventive, and excitingly geared to the development of human potential.

The authors of the emerging model described below suggest that what is required will be a period of testing, modification, and blending with the conceptualizations of other educators, student personnel workers, faculty and administrators "who believe in and who have begun to provide opportunities for the full development of human potential" (O'Banion, Thurston, and Gulden, 1970). The writers believe that this model is an excellent one for faculty and staff in nursing programs, especially those in diploma schools, for it directly relates to difficulties and problems the latter group are facing and may provide insight on dealing with changing student attitudes. Considering the professional role and functions of nurses, the model which emphasizes human development should be especially appealing. Throughout the remainder of this chapter, advisors will be referred to as facilitators, who could be faculty in diploma schools as well as student personnel staff in two- or four-year colleges with whom nursing students may have contact.

A human development facilitator not only deals with students but also facilitates the development of all the groups in an educational community—faculty, administrators, nonacademic workers, and even the board members. Facilitate, it is suggested, "is an encountering verb which means to free, to make way for, to open the door to," and whether the human development facilitator is a counselor or a faculty member, she must

> be committed to positive human development; . . . possess the skills and the expertise that will enable . . . (her) to implement programs for the realization of human potential; . . . be able to communicate with administrators in the college; and . . . be able to keep the functions and services under . . . (her) responsibility operating efficiently (and effectively). (O'Banion, Thurston, and Gulden, 1970.)

Fundamental to the emerging model "is a belief that man is a growing organism, capable of moving toward self-fulfillment and responsible social development and whose potential for both has been only partially realized." There are, according to its authors, implications of climate—a climate of learning—and outcome. There is a behavioral orientation to a student development point of view. A "climate of learning" must provide students the freedom to choose their own directions for learning as well as the responsibility for their choices. Student interpersonal interaction with a learning facilitator should include challenge, encounter, stimulation, confrontation, and excitement—not the usual, often dull, interplay between a student and an advisor; it should demonstrate warmth, caring, understanding, and acceptance—characteristics of a supportive counseling relationship; and it should demonstrate an appreciation of individual differences.

A facilitator must accept students "where they are at," regardless of differences, in a "nonjudgmental" manner. The latter suggests simply an ability to deal with all kinds of students with all sorts of problems and differences.

"Through such a facilitative atmosphere," the authors of the new model suggest, "the outcomes of student development would be increased in:

1. Intellectual understanding
2. Skill competencies

3. Socially responsible behavior
4. Flexibility and creativity
5. Awareness of self and others
6. Acceptance of self and others
7. Courage to explore and experiment
8. Openness to experience
9. Efficient and effective ability to learn
10. Ability to respond positively to change
11. A useful value system
12. A satisfying life style.

Facilitators are expected to be committed to humanistic values, and to be aware of the changing values of man as offered by Tannenbaum and Davis (1969), who suggest that

> Man, perhaps to an extent greater than ever before, is coming alive; he is ceasing to be an object to be used and is increasingly asserting himself, his complexity, and his importance. Not quite understanding why or how, he is moving slowly but ever closer to the center of the universe.

We are in a period of transition during which Tannenbaum and Davis (1969) suggest our view of man moving

> away from avoidance or negative evaluation of individuals toward basically good;

> away from avoidance or negative evaluation of individuals towards confirming them as human beings;

> away from viewing individuals as fixed, toward viewing them as being in process;

> away from resisting and fearing individual differences toward acceptance and utilization of the differences;

> away from the utilization of an individual primarily with reference to his role—as a student, a worker, and so forth—toward viewing him as a whole person;

> away from walling-off the expression of feelings toward valuing possibly both appropriate expression and effective use;

> away from maskmanship and game-playing toward authentic behavior;

> away from distrusting humans toward trusting them; and

> away from avoidance of risk-taking toward willingness to risk.

A *human development facilitator* must view every student as a gifted person possessing untapped potentialities who is capable of much fuller life. He or she must be "interested in all students, in helping those who are unhealthy to become more healthy, and in helping those who are already healthy to achieve yet ever greater health" (O'Banion, Thurston, and Gulden, 1970).

Those responsible for student development in the diploma institutions, or those responsible in two-year or four-year institutions for out-of-class advisement to nursing students, should strive to provide an open climate—a facilitative atmosphere—for this, as suggested, has prime implications for the student development program. A significant factor in the proper climate relates to the rules and regulations which prevail in the institutional setting and are applicable to nursing students.

## RULES AND REGULATIONS

We would suggest that rules and regulations be based only on the infringement upon the rights of others. Constant review is the key to rules and regulations which are applicable to current societal attitudes and the hypocritical regulation which implies an attitude of *in loco parentis* with overtones of control which do not encourage student growth and development.

Joseph Fordyce (1969) suggests:

> First, limit the scope of regulations to really important matters. Second, scrap the whole body of regulations periodically and begin with a new set as it is needed. Third, make them say what they mean and help everyone in the institution to understand that they mean what they say.

Rigid rules and regulations based on personal value systems and idiosyncrasies of faculty or staff rather than pertinent matters, and with the involvement and input of students (those to be regulated), tend to be negative, irrelevant, and hypocritical as well as completely meaningless and unenforceable. Such rules and regulations can only lead to frustration, anxiety, dishonesty, and often rebellion on the part of students. Mary M. Meluskey, discussing student relations at the 12th Annual Workshop for Faculties of Schools of Nursing held at Penn State University during the summer of 1971, listed the following kinds of rules and regulations as some that "bug" students:

1. Those with no logical reason
2. Unwritten regulations
3. Overprotective regulations
4. Room inspections
5. Regulations which include words like: moderate, appropriate, sparingly, in good taste, and so forth
6. Regulations which govern behavior in locations outside the school.

Meluskey raised the following questions:
Should we try to be moral disciplinarians?
Can we honestly justify our rules and regulations as being necessary?

Do we find the habits of students as being contrary to our own moral values?

Further questions about the validity of regulations were offered as to curfew restrictions, dress regulations, quiet hours, demerit systems, part-time jobs, married and pregnant students, restrictions on where students can go, and so forth.

Meluskey further states that "rules and regulations should be reviewed yearly," but we would suggest that review dates be scheduled more often if students desire such or if they present valid evidence for evaluation. Additionally, rules "should be helping rather than punitive," positive rather than negative, with the growth and development of the students being governed always kept in mind.

A facilitator should function as the "guardian against the oppressive regulations that tend to develop without question in most institutions." Traditional educational trappings such as "probation and suspension regulations, F grades, social probation, dress codes, (and) regulations regarding work load . . . may hinder the development of human potential more than they help." If facilitators are concerned about student development, they justifiably should assist students in ferreting out the repressive philosophy that supports unwarranted rules and regulations, especially if they are to assist in developing what O'Banion, Thurston, and Gulden (1970) call "a total institutional climate conducive to the development of human potential." Nevertheless, faculty or staff functioning as facilitators must do so within a sound rationale so as not to be viewed as "standard wreckers" by faculty.

As to standards, Meluskey (1971) suggests:

> There has been an erosion in discipline in the home and in school. We cannot be *in loco parentis* and usurp the real parental role. Once we stop trying to be standard bearers and upholders of virtue then we can become teachers and innovators.

## STUDENTS' RIGHTS AND FREEDOMS

Within a climate of learning it is only logical to assume that students' freedom to pursue their own directions is a fundamental right guaranteed by the Constitution of the United States. Many statements have been developed in recent years on student freedoms, including a "Joint Statement on Rights and Freedoms of Students" prepared in 1967 by the American Association of University Professors, National Student Association, Association of American Colleges, National Association of Student Personnel Administrators, and National Association of Women Deans and Counselors. This statement can be found in its entirety in the Appendix.

On June 14, 1966, at the American Nurses' Association Convention in San Francisco, Dorothy Mereness (1967) presented her views on student freedoms in a paper entitled "Freedom and Responsibility for Nursing Students." Mereness suggested that nursing had developed few practitioners who could think critically and imaginatively or solve problems in unique, constructive ways. Nurses rather tend to accept things as they are and to conform to the situation.

Mereness (1967) listed six freedoms and responsibilities which she felt students had a right to expect in any educational institution:

| *Freedom* | *Responsibility* |
|---|---|
| 1. To disagree | 1. To identify respectfully reasons for disagreement |
| 2. To explore new ideas | 2. To evaluate fairly the old and new |
| 3. To help choose one's educational goals and patterns | 3. To use advisor's wisdom, society's needs, and one's personal aspirations |
| 4. To study independently | 4. To pursue a significant purpose and invest time wisely |
| 5. To experiment with alternate methods | 5. To define purpose, expected outcomes, and necessary steps |
| 6. To know faculty members as human beings | 6. To allow relationship to be mutually beneficial |

The Student Nurses' Association of Illinois have written a Student Bill of Rights (1969) in which they outline rights and freedoms for nurses under categories titled Personal Rights, Academic Rights, Participatory Democracy, and Rights of Due Process. The Participatory Democracy section states that within student affairs the following standards must be maintained if student freedom is to be maintained:

> 1. Student government shall be free of faculty control and shall have full power to set policies respecting matters of student concern.
> As to advisers, each organization should have the freedom to choose its own and the inability to choose an adviser should not result in the withholding or withdrawing of institutional recognition.
> 2. Students and student organizations should be free to examine and to discuss all questions of interest to them, and to express opinions publicly and privately. This includes supporting causes by orderly means which do not disrupt regular and/or essential operation of the institution.
> 3. Students should be free to invite speakers of their own choice and neither "routine procedures" for registering an event nor institutional control of campus facilities should be used as a device of censorship. It should be made clear to all, faculty and the larger community, that sponsorship of a speaker does not represent endorsement or necessarily imply approval of views expressed by the speaker, either by the sponsoring group or the institution.

Again the emphasis is upon the provision of an open climate in which students are allowed to plan, promote, and carry out activities with full responsibility for their actions without the need for an advisor's approval on every detail of an event or even final approval. A facilitator's role then becomes one of encouraging students to pursue free inquiry and free expression. In this way, facilitators truly will be assisting each student to explore the dimensions of potential development rather than forcing students to follow directions or to conform rigidly to detailed rules and regulations, which are often set up to protect outdated concepts.

Though considerable emphasis in all bills of rights is placed upon procedural standards in conduct or disciplinary proceedings, space will not allow treatment in this discussion. The reader is referred to an excellent treatment of both the old and new points of view on disciplinary administration in the Academic section of the Handbook of College and University Administration (Bowers and Salem, 1970).

Recently a six-member Task Force on College and University Governance of Commission IV of the American College Personnel Association issued a proposed statement on student participation in the governance of higher educational institutions. It was proposed that students have primary responsibility for determination of standards of student conduct "for the formulation of standards and regulations pertaining to their personal conduct" on those campuses where separate student conduct codes are in existence. Additionally, primary responsibility should prevail for the establishment of procedures that govern student discipline, because, since

> discipline, as well as standards of student conduct, help determine the tone and quality of the total environment, faculty and administration are concerned and must be involved. However, students should be given maximum control within institution policies. (McKaig, 1971.)

Throughout their experiences with students and student organizations, facilitators must remember that students are guaranteed their rights by the Constitution of the United States and that students today are much more aware of their rights through all forms of media, especially television. Student personnel workers in colleges have always worked with young, developing adults, but far too often, either owing to their personal attitudes or as a result of top administration attitudes, advisors have treated college students as irresponsible kids.

In the very near future, as a consequence of the lowering of the voting age to 18 years, all states will probably make 18 the majority age. It has occurred in Michigan at this date and is about to do so in many other states. This gives even more significance to the new model outlined above which suggests that student development, rather than control, should be the prime function, not only of those acting as facilitators, but also of all members of the faculty and administration. Facilitators must encourage students to become involved in their own activity programs as well as in the total institution.

The burden of establishing an atmosphere of freedom which is conducive to a climate of learning falls upon all staff and faculty, for, as O'Banion, Thurston, and Gulden (1970) suggest, the human development facilitator must work with not only students, but faculty and other staff as well. Facilitators can extend the impact of their program by becoming involved in academic departments in terms of their own background and interests, by becoming acquainted with faculty to improve communication, and by assisting and encouraging students in the development of discipline-related activities.

The Student Nurses' Association of Illinois in their Student Bill of Rights also suggest that faculty and staff have equal responsibility in providing an open climate; i.e. the responsibility to secure and to respect general conditions necessary to guarantee freedom to learn should be shared by all members of the academic community. They also state that "each school of nursing has a duty to develop policies and procedures which provide and safeguard this freedom."

## STUDENT INVOLVEMENT

> There has been a great hesitance to involve students in major decision-making processes. Yet it would appear students have had a marked influence on American higher education, regardless of their lack of legitimate power; they have profoundly affected the curriculum and the extracurriculum. What they are now demanding, therefore, appears to be the right to influence the university in more positive and effective ways. (Fleming, 1969.)

An excellent example of nursing students' ability to carry out positive and responsible action was described by Ryder and Wilson (1969). The administration and faculty of the Los Angeles City College Department of Nursing had been unable to convince college administrators of the need for accreditation by the National League for Nursing. With the permission of the chairman of the Nursing department, a student discussed the matter with the president of the college and arranged a meeting of college administrators and nursing students. After this, students collected money to pay for accreditation visits, collected materials pertaining to the State Board's position on accreditation, gathered reports from students who had left the school because government assistance was unavailable without NLN accreditation, and developed evidence that other schools had special accreditation within six months.

At Rutgers, the State University of New Jersey, Newark campus, students in the University College of Nursing staged a mild revolt. The students called for a mass meeting with their faculty at which they presented two demands which they wanted fulfilled within one week: one third representation on all faculty committees plus an advisory program to be established for all students. Additionally, the nursing students wanted the school to recruit more black students as well as black faculty. The response to the demands included changes in the committee membership, a faculty-student committee to work on assisting students from minority groups to enroll in nursing, and an investigation toward implementing a counseling program (Mildrow, 1969).

Unfortunately the actions of students that are made public are too often those in which "confrontation" brings about change. We believe that the reason for many confrontations is that administrators and faculty often react too slowly or not at all until threatened.

Students can and do make worthwhile contributions to our programs. So why not commit ourselves to assist them in developing and carrying out programs toward alleviating conditions not appropriate to a climate of learning? When we consider the quick response given to demands after they are made through confrontation, we must question the reason for procrastination on the part of administration and faculty prior to the demands. It is better to act than react, and far too many actions on the part of those in charge are reactions.

## STUDENT HOUSING

Colleges and universities have been considering different types of living-learning arrangements in residence halls for some time, because they suggest that students have different life styles and that the opportunity to choose from alternatives must be available. Choices may encompass halls with no-hour policies and those with curfews; those with no visitation and those with 24-hour privileges; those with freshmen clustered together and those mixing with other students; and those with graduate students living with upperclassmen as well as those separate from all undergraduate students. Groupings are provided on the basis of academically interested students such as high scholarship or in tutorial groups. Single-room accommodations as well as personal choice of roommates are also part of the freedoms in choice now offered students, especially on larger campuses.

Many colleges have discarded the idea that older women should function as house mothers so that both undergraduate and graduate students can earn money working as resident advisors or counselors and resident directors. No longer is the concept of *in loco parentis* valid, yet Wilson (1970) suggests that the faculty in the diploma school may have a tendency to function in this manner.

> Consider, for example, the way in which a (nursing) student exchanged the physical dependence of her home for that of the residence (in the diploma), with its time tables and house rules. Even the common adolescent daughter-mother conflict is in danger of perpetuation, as authority figures in nursing seek to counsel and correct the student on matters of her personal life and appearance.

The subjective complaints of nursing students, according to Wilson, dealt with loss of individuality, the exhaustive concentration on nursing, and constriction of students' interests. Nursing students also viewed nursing as a dull and frustrating profession from which it was impossible to break free because of investments of time, money, and effort. The only solution left to the frustrated and bored students was escape from hospital practice after graduation.

Wilson found that student contacts were primarily with other nurses, and the students had come to believe that nursing consisted merely in the execution of routine, physical tasks. They complained of living in the

school residence, eating in the hospital cafeteria, and being subject to instructors, counselors, and directors, all of whom were nurses—a sort of
intense concentration which can breed not only revolt, but also a staleness
and the constriction of interests mentioned above. All these contribute
to the problem of student attrition.

Other professions, except for the religious and the military, no longer
segregate their novices because cloisterization frustrates legitimate
emotional tasks which during personality development are appropriate
to a student's age and maturity. The primary task of the adolescent is
to find her own unique identity, but according to Wilson, "the traditional
structure of nursing education, community living, and the demands of
role formation . . . fail to provide what the adolescent needs for . . .
(personal) maturation." In actuality these conditions frustrate the process of self-discovery "by encouraging nonmaturing psychic activities."

As far as the teaching process is concerned, emphasis has always been
on the classroom, whereas the learning process is viewed as an ongoing
process occurring in a variety of places over 24 hours a day. With the
growing interest in learning as an ongoing process, educators are finally
becoming concerned about the living habitat of their students, whether
on or off campus (Riker, 1970).

Learning, Riker states, as do others who espouse the development
of a learning climate, an open climate, or atmosphere of freedom, is an
individualistic matter. Each person determines what she hears and what
has meaning for her. But there are a number of conditions which influence her decisions: her associations with others; the atmosphere of acceptance and security in which ideas can be examined informally; her
readiness for learning; and the environment, both physical and social.

A student's living group is a social environment which can exert
significant control over a member's goals and values. It also influences
her attitudes toward the educational institution, its programs, and the
quality of participation (Riker, 1970). For example, Wilson (1970) found
that nursing students felt the cloistered situation less influential than the
school in having a significant bearing on their life style. Students were
disturbed "about their failure to continue reading to keep up with the
news, and to maintain interest in the movements, styles and causes of
the day." They also "complained about boredom and the apparent super-
human effort it takes to break out of such a community." The freedom
to choose their own direction was lacking from the inception of their
program, and it became less feasible as it progressed.

Student responses, according to Wilson, were not necessarily limited
to Canadian institutions in Toronto, since he had heard complaints
similar in content, tone, and intensity in Atlanta, Georgia, and Richmond,
Virginia, schools. He believes that there is a consistency related to
cloisterization which "has been a traditional and integral part of nursing
education." He suggests that the

> aspects of the system against which students react are seen as essential
> and integral parts of the structure of that education by those that gov-
> ern it. . . . (In nursing schools) both students and educators agree that
> what we are talking about does exist. (But) in a student's eyes it is a

heavy burden, in an educator's it is seen as part of the ethos of the whole enterprise.

What recommendations can be made? Wilson's suggestions on nursing education are comparable to those recommended by O'Banion, Thurston, and Gulden on education in general. Wilson feels that pressure should be brought to make structural changes in nursing education which will permit not only personal freedom, but also individual responsibility and accountability. He proposes several recommendations which affect different aspects of a student's involvement with an educational structure, all of which he feels would be of equal significance to her.

1. Provide the opportunity to live either outside the hospital environment or within residences with students and practitioners of other schools or disciplines based in the hospital.

2. Management of student residences should be independent of the school of nursing and the administration.

3. Students should manage their own finances, including the renegotiating of their grants and loans rather than the method of providing room, meals, and tuition without presentation of any account.

4. Students should be allowed and encouraged to work in the hospital or school to help finance their education.

Further recommendations pertaining to occupational choice, curriculum, and respect for student performance rather than attitude were made by Wilson.

Above all, Wilson seems to be suggesting freedom of choice for nursing students much the same as others are suggesting for all students. Depending on their circumstances and their urban location, diploma schools should evaluate their policies and procedures to determine whether or not they may be stultifying students' growth and development. Facilitators also should attempt to make other faculty aware of possible infringements on the rights of their students.

## STUDENT ACTIVITIES

Nursing students attending two- and four-year colleges should have few difficulties finding or developing activities in which they may participate if their academic schedules allow time for involvement. A more difficult situation faces nursing students in diploma schools—difficulties which relate to limitations imposed by residence, by *in loco parentis* attitudes of faculty and staff and by schedules which leave little time to pursue outside or other interests.

Again an emphasis on freedom to pursue their own interests should be the key to resolving problems to the development of meaningful programs. Students, not faculty or staff, should determine the what, when, where, how, and why of their activity programs, and the facilitator should function as an advocate and a resource person by interpretation to faculty and by providing assistance to students when requested.

Student activities programs can be social, recreational, educational, cultural, and political, or a combination of all. Perhaps the only limitations will be availability of resources, especially money and physical facilities in a diploma school. Diploma schools located in urban communities should seek cooperative arrangements with public or community center organizations which contain facilities students may use for recreational or other purposes.

Student activities have a tendency to become traditional and archaic. The archaic aspect may be a consequence of faculty and staff attitudes rather than of student desires. Recognition and acceptance of temporary activities should prevail in all higher education institutions to allow students and student groups to be spontaneous, creative, and innovative. Often, though, elaborate, bureaucratic methods of organizational recognition preclude temporary activities. A facilitator should function as an advocate in assisting students to change outdated or *in loco parentis* policies and procedures which exist to control or forestall nontraditional student activities. As suggested by Bloland (1970), it is "good institutional practice to keep . . . (regulations and policies) to an absolute minimum and to establish procedures whereby such policies and regulations can be quickly reviewed and revised in the light of changing circumstances."

Recent student interest in significant campus, community, and societal affairs offers innumerable opportunities for student growth and development through activities which have educational implications, such as community volunteer and tutorial services, as well as involvement in the governing and administrative structure of their schools.

Not all learning takes place in classes, as we are all aware. Activity programs can provide not only learning experiences but also tension-relieving projects, but faculty determine the kind and direction of programs. Students must develop their own projects, and they will. Meluskey (1971) stated that students at the National Student Nurses' Association Convention "went on record as to their intent to become more involved in community projects." This is understandable, according to Meluskey, who continues:

> Students are city-bred, and they will continue to live in the city. Students want more involvement in the city. . . . Getting good grades is not the only way one learns. . . . Projects may relate to cultural enrichment, tutorial sessions, social work, community action, or the drug abuse program.

Meluskey recommends that the orientation program for nursing students must have input from students or it will likely be a bore. Students can do a better job of explaining rules and regulations, especially if they were involved in setting up the rules as suggested above.

Nursing students, whether in a two-, three- or four-year college, should be involved in the college life. And the facilitator can assist students to explore new alternatives for involvement, such as "special task forces, ad hoc groups, town meetings." Where the traditional committee structure is utilized,

> students should be on all the committees of the college. This should extend far beyond the old worn-out student government association

in which students play sandbox government and spend their time quarreling over student activity fee allocations. (O'Banion, Thurston, and Gulden, 1970.)

Serving on committees does not necessarily mean the curriculum committee or one on faculty evaluation. It also means the main administrative council and even the board of trustees. But if students are involved to this extent, a facilitator should be aware of "academic and bureaucratic dynamics" so that she may educate students on the best methods of functioning effectively while serving as contributing members of committees (O'Banion, Thurston, and Gulden, 1970).

New and creative learning experiences are available to students when functioning as paraprofessionals, and the "means of getting students involved in the education of other students" must be a concern of the facilitator's, for she, through contact and association with other faculty, can constantly strive to develop an awareness of the significance of student activities as additional learning opportunities. Also, she can solicit interested faculty who are ready and willing to cooperate in an effort to provide these experiences for students (O'Banion, Thurston, and Gulden, 1970).

## STUDENT GOVERNMENT

This chapter does not offer the opportunity to go into detail about kinds of student government, which range from the traditional model which usually exists with a faculty senate and from which many other forms emanate, to the all-college or all-university senate model in which governance of the institution is jointly exercised by both constituencies, and the administration serves as an executive body approving ideas and proposals as well as implementation of finalized policies. Rather, the reader is referred to an article in the *Junior College Journal* entitled "Student Participation in Governance," in which the American Association of Junior Colleges Student Personnel Commission described various methods of involving students in the policy-making decisions of colleges (Deegan, Drexel, Collins, and Kearney, 1970).

Educators and students alike are aware of the fact that student governments in most colleges and universities have become meaningless governing bodies, for they are viewed as powerless by a majority of students, lack real authority, represent elective processes that generally are popularity contests in which few students participate, and, once elected, spend the majority of their time quibbling over procedural matters. Given these problems, nursing student facilitators in two- and four-year colleges may find it difficult to encourage nursing students to become active in a student governing association.

Yet on most campuses it is the student government which has the power to allocate their own funds as derived from student activity fees, and representation may be required to secure monies for student nurse association programs—such as speakers, workshops, films, orientation, volunteer services, and the like.

As far as diploma schools are concerned, it should be obvious that nursing students should control their own activity-fee monies and determine how these monies will be spent. Add to this the foregoing recommendations about housing, rules and regulations, and orientation programs, and nursing students may well feel that they control at least one phase of their destiny. If a facilitator can also educate other faculty members as to the educational value of student control over their own affairs as well as participation in the academic affairs of the school, then she will be assisting in the development of human potential, i.e. the human potential which in the very near future will be making the professional decisions in conjunction with students, for all nurses.

# Chapter 15

# *Student Personnel Services: Program Evaluation*

Throughout this book we have been presenting information about the guidance, counseling, and student personnel program in schools of nursing. We have also made a number of recommendations about specific phases of the overall program. These recommendations are an extension of the stated criteria by the National League for Nursing in 1969; i.e. "policies for health services and counseling and guidance services are provided and implemented." Yet no matter how carefully and thoroughly a comprehensive program of student services is developed, it is important that the program be regularly evaluated to determine its effectiveness and whether it still meets the current needs of the school. This process of continuous program research and evaluation is frequently overlooked under the constant pressures of conducting a program. As a result, a good deal of educational planning is a result of crisis management rather than systematic planning, i.e. looking closely at each phase of the program only when the need arises, rather than regularly and comprehensively reviewing all phases.

The purpose of this chapter is to explore several of the ways that program evaluation can be conducted, using as examples several evaluative studies done in recent years. From the outset it must be recognized that problems in evaluation will differ among the various nursing programs, and that our objective should be to make evaluation relevant to the particular school and its needs. We have at various points in the book suggested specific ways of evaluating specific phases of an overall program. At this point we are primarily interested in the broad evaluation process for an entire program, rather than just for one aspect or activity. A well done evaluation can greatly facilitate program revision, and help to ensure that the student personnel services program continues to fulfill the objectives of the school, and the needs and concerns of the student body.

## CRITERIA FOR PROGRAM EVALUATION

Perhaps the main problem that arises in program evaluation lies in the ambiguity or lack of any established criteria. Without some agreement on criteria, program evaluation ends up as little more than the subjective opinion of one or more people. Fortunately, we have at least the beginnings of legitimate criteria. To start with, the National League for

*216*

Nursing in 1971 made certain recommendations as to what should be included in a comprehensive guidance and counseling program for diploma schools. The recommendations are as follows:

The guidance services should include personal, professional, and academic counseling. Responsibility for the development of objectives and policies for these services rests with the faculty. The direction and coordination of the services must be clearly defined. Some schools employ qualified guidance counselors on a full-time or part-time basis, and these persons carry out the major part of the guidance activities. In such instances, however, faculty members continue to fulfill guidance responsibilities related to the role of instructor. If a qualified counselor is not employed, faculty members must assume major responsibility for meeting the students' counseling and guidance needs. It is also the faculty's responsibility to create an environment that supports the objectives of the counseling and guidance services, and the plan of implementation should include conferences initiated by faculty or students. Provision should be made for referral of students with problems to appropriate specialists—skilled counselors, psychiatrists, psychologists, or religious advisors—for personal or professional guidance. The school and the cooperating agencies should make provision for the exchange of pertinent information regarding the counseling of students. The guidance records should include pre-admission data as well as information regarding the students' use of the services. The confidential aspect of the counseling and guidance process should be respected and maintained by all school personnel.

These recommendations of the NLN serve as a useful guideline for all schools of nursing, not just diploma schools, but they need to be translated into practice in order to determine program effectiveness. All the services described may be provided, and yet the program may still not be effectively serving the needs of students. Rackham (1951) developed perhaps the most comprehensive method for evaluating student personnel programs and services. Rackham's Student Personnel Services Inventory was designed to assist colleges and universities in evaluating their programs of student personnel services. As he comments, "It should be obvious that such programs of student personnel services activities ought to be subjected periodically to a thorough review so that needed adjustments can be identified and given proper attention."

The Rackham Inventory was originally constructed by combining the efforts of 381 personnel officers from 113 colleges and universities who participated by reviewing lists of tentative criteria in the areas of their specialization. They were asked to check the comprehensiveness of the lists, and to determine whether each statement was satisfactory or unsatisfactory in terms of the "ideal" student personnel services program for the "average" American college or university. The resulting scale was then weighted by ten experts in the field of student personnel services. The present form of the Inventory includes over 800 questions, and is designed to allow a school or college to compare its program with the ideal standards as viewed by experts in each field. Those schools that have only selected student personnel services can use only selected portions of the Inventory.

An outline of the topical headings in the Inventory will help the reader see the comprehensive nature of the instrument.

A. Admissions
   1. Some general considerations
   2. Legislative and executive considerations
   3. Types of information upon which admission is based
   4. Utilization of a combination of factors
B. Counseling
   1. Some general considerations
   2. Who should be counseled
   3. Levels of counseling
      a. The lay level
      b. The semi-professional level
      c. The professional level
   4. General techniques and sources of data
   5. Major types of student problems
      a. Educational counseling
      b. Vocational counseling
      c. Personal counseling
   6. Evidences of effectiveness of a counseling program
C. Discipline
   1. Basic assumptions behind a disciplinary program
   2. Organization and administration of discipline
D. Extra-curricular activities
   1. The need for extra-curricular activities
   2. Penalties
   3. Range of activities
   4. Extent of participation
E. Financial aid
   1. Some general considerations
   2. Scholarships, grants-in-aid, loans, part-time employment
   3. Organization and administration of financial aid
F. Health service
   1. The need and importance of a health service
   2. Physical and medical examinations
   3. Clinical and infirmary services
   4. Informational program for personal and community health
   5. Applied program for personal and community health
   6. Public health program
   7. Organization and administration
G. Housing and board
   1. Some general considerations
   2. Types of housing afforded students
   3. Organization and administration
H. Organization and administration (general)
I. Orientation
   1. Some general considerations
   2. Examinations and tests
   3. Group meetings
J. Placement
   1. Some general considerations
   2. Records
   3. Making occupational information available to students
   4. Organization and administration of placement services
K. Pre-College counseling
   1. Some general considerations
   2. Need for proper articulation between institutions

    3. Means which are employed by institutions of higher learning to
       contact prospective students
L. Records
    1. The need for adequate records
    2. Desirable information for records
    3. Organization and administration of records
M. Religion
    1. Some general considerations
    2. Organization and administration of campus religious program
    3. Religious counseling
N. Research
    1. Some general considerations
    2. Needed research
O. Testing
    1. Some general considerations
    2. Administration of the testing program
    3. Some uses of test results

The Rackham Student Personnel Services Inventory is a useful instrument for use in part or as a whole in evaluating programs. Readers may also be interested in the work of Hage (1957), who constructed a revision of the Rackham Inventory with less than 400 items. Both these instruments are worth close examination by those charged with the responsibility for evaluating all phases of a student personnel services program.

Metzler (1964) surveyed the literature on the evaluation of counseling and guidance programs. In the course of his survey he made three observations:

1. There is no agreement as to what constitutes the goals of a guidance program, and therefore it is impossible to determine criteria to measure effectiveness.

2. Current research to determine the effectiveness of programs is of little value

3. Expert judgment and opinion are the primary acceptable criteria by which we measure counselor and program effectiveness.

Metzler feels that two things are needed before effective evaluation of guidance and counseling programs can be made. First, there needs to be a decision as to what constitutes proper criteria. Second, strong emphasis needs to be placed on longitudinal studies to determine program effectiveness.

Litwack et al. (1968) spoke of the problem of evaluating counseling effectiveness. They stated:

> A major reason for the difficulty in conducting research on counseling lies in the inability to arrive at satisfactory criteria of success. Most research into counseling falls short of being definitive because the criteria usually amount to little more than a value judgment implicit in an instrument or on what happens to the counselee after counseling which is assumed to be desirable.

The same principles apply to the entire student personnel program, rather than to just the counseling services provided. For example, even though the Rackham Inventory delineates a number of important areas, the success of its application will still depend largely on the expert judgment and opinion suggested by Metzler.

## PARTICIPANTS IN THE EVALUATION PROCESS

A great many of the problems in the evaluation process arise from the fact that all those who should be actively involved in evaluation are seldom included. In some instances only a small group of persons are asked to give their opinion about the relative merits of the various aspects of a guidance, counseling, and student personnel program. Such selectivity does little to ensure that a representative cross section of opinions is gathered about the various program phases. In order to provide a complete, representative, and reasonably accurate picture of the effects of any program, it is desirable to obtain data from five sources: faculty members, students, graduates, withdrawals and terminations, and employers. Each of these provides a valuable dimension in understanding all the possible ramifications of a program.

Faculty members need to be actively involved in the evaluation process. Through the use of questionnaires, rating scales, check lists, anecdotal material, self-report instruments, and so forth, information needs to be gathered as to their perceptions of what services are provided to students, and how effective they believe these services to be. It is not sufficient, however, to rely solely on written reports. In order to increase the validity of the information gathered, it is essential that structured interviews be conducted among at least a random sample of the faculty to verify the information gathered in written form. By maintaining the anonymity of both written and interview data, increased validity and reliability can be obtained. This occurs because some faculty members are inevitably hesitant about criticizing aspects of a program that they have developed, and for which they have a large responsibility.

It is essential for students to be involved in the process of program evaluation, for they, after all, are the *raison d'etre* for the program's existence. As the consumer of the services provided, their judgments and attitudes toward those services are of vital importance in determining the worth and effectiveness of each facet of the program. Ideally, a survey should be conducted at the end of each year among at least a representative sample of the student body. Through use of the same techniques as with the faculty, information can be gathered as to students' perceptions of personnel, services provided, additional program needs, and the like. Such information will serve as a validity check on the perceptions of the faculty. As we discussed in Part 1, even if faculty members perceive certain services as available to students, if the students do not feel that these services are available or worthwhile, then consideration must immediately be given to a revision or correction of the apparent program deficiencies.

The third group that needs to be surveyed are the recent graduates from the school of nursing. This can be done just prior to graduation, and a follow-up conducted six months to a year after graduation. Having successfully completed the educational program of the school, the graduates are able to review objectively the services provided by the school, and their effectiveness. The inherent limitation to surveying graduates is that their responses tend to be dependent on their memory. If a survey is made of the previous year's graduates, however, the results should be reasonably accurate and meaningful. Again, the same techniques may be used in obtaining the reactions of the graduates as those previously described for the faculty and students. It may not always be possible to utilize structured interviews, but all other procedures are applicable. Among other things, graduates should be asked to describe what they feel were the strong points and the areas that should be improved for each facet of the total student personnel program.

Those students who leave the school for any reason prior to graduation also need to be interviewed. Of all groups, this one is perhaps the most important, for it may reflect the failure or the inadequacies of the student personnel program. At least theoretically, those students who withdrew, who failed and were terminated, and who transferred out could have been maintained successfully in school if the guidance counseling and student personnel programs had been able to fulfill their functions to the highest degree. These students should be asked to identify the services of the school of which they were aware, those services that were used, and reactions to those that were used. In addition, this group should be asked why they did not use services provided by the school or college. Perhaps the best time to survey this group of students would be as part of the exit process just prior to their leaving the school. A follow-up interview or report should also be obtained later, for students' feelings tend to run high prior to leaving, particularly if they feel negative. These same principles can be applied to students by counselors both prior to their leaving and as a follow-up.

The final group that should be reviewed would include the employers of the graduates from the school and the professional personnel outside the school of nursing who come into constant contact with the students. This group cannot legitimately be asked to comment on the specific facets of a student personnel program, for they will generally be unaware of details. They are, however, able to relate the kinds of problems presented by the students or graduates, and give their professional reactions as to ways these problems might be alleviated or prevented.

As we have tried to emphasize consistently throughout this book, the educational program of a school of nursing is only as good as the various elements that are part of it, and the creativity of those responsible for developing it. Just as everyone has a stake in the educational program, so does everyone have a vital stake in the effectiveness of the student personnel program which serves it. To emphasize this combined responsibility, all the groups described above have something to contribute in developing a comprehensive program, and should be involved in the continual evaluation of the student personnel program.

## EXAMPLES OF EVALUATION STUDIES

In the previous section we described the various groups that should be involved in the evaluation of the guidance, counseling, and student personnel program. At this point it would be useful to examine several studies that exemplify different methods of program evaluation. These studies are not meant to serve as models for future evaluations, but rather as the stimulus for the creative development of new and improved evaluation techniques.

Kaback (1958), in the process of developing a manual on guidance and counseling, sent a questionnaire to 48 schools of nursing throughout the country that were members of the Council of Member Agencies of the Department of Diploma and Associate Degree Programs of the National League for Nursing, asking for the cooperation of faculty and students in a study on "Guidance Services and Counseling Needs in Schools of Nursing." Forty-four schools agreed to cooperate. Out of a total of 4274 questionnaire forms which were mailed out, 1944, or 45 per cent, were returned from 40 of the original 44 schools. These included 1468 first-, second-, and third-year students, 84 administrators, 210 instructors, and 182 nursing service personnel who described the various guidance and counseling activities developed in their schools, and offered recommendations for improving them.

Although the return was much lower than would have been desired, the distribution of the questionnaires covered four of the five groups that we discussed in the previous section. The Kaback study was not designed to evaluate a specific program within a specific school of nursing. The techniques used, however, are illustrative of the sort of comprehensive survey studies that are needed if we hope to improve our student personnel programs.

The questionnaire developed by Kaback serves as a useful beginning example for future evaluation studies. It included a careful explanation of the rationale for the study, specific directions, and the questionnaire itself. The following is part of the questionnaire used:

Study on Guidance Services and
Counseling Needs in Schools of Nursing

*Reasons for Study*
There has been a good deal of discussion regarding the need for more guidance and counseling services in schools of nursing. Faculties are concerned that many guidance and counseling programs fall short of their stated objectives. There is considerable feeling that this may be due, at least in part, to the fact that the consumers (the nursing students), faculty members, and other staff members have not had an opportunity to participate in the formulation of plans for their particular programs. In sponsoring the present study, the NLN is hopeful of developing plans for giving more assistance to schools in this area of guidance and counseling and believes that members of the nursing profession should have an opportunity to assist with the blueprinting of plans for the anticipated guidance and counseling services.

*Directions*
Let us assume that you have been invited to become a member of a committee concerned with the organization of guidance and counseling services for your school of nursing and with the selection of those who will act as counselors. It is expected that these counselors will

assist nursing students and others with problems which they might want to bring to them. In your role of committee members, will you answer the following questions using the reverse side of the sheet as necessary? Be assured that your remarks will be held in strictest confidence.

1. What kind of educational training would you expect the counselor to have? Why?
2. What kind of professional experience would you expect the counselor to have had? Why?
3. Do you think that the counselor should have teaching or administrative duties in addition to counseling responsibilities? Why, or why not?
4. What problems would you personally bring to this counselor? Why?
5. What kind of help would you expect to receive from this counselor? Why?
6. What kind of assistance would you be able to give this counselor? Why?
7. What kind of person would you suggest for the position of counselor? Why?
8. What other factors do you consider important? Why?
9. Describe the major limitations of your present guidance and counseling service. How do you think these limitations might be overcome?
10. Describe the major values of your present guidance and counseling service. How might these values be extended?

The Kaback report serves as a useful example of a large-scale survey study. Even though the questionnaire could be improved by being more specific, the conclusions drawn would be well worth reading by all those concerned with the development of guidance and counseling programs.

Ludwig (1968) provides an example of a study designed to look at one specific aspect of a guidance and counseling program. She was interested in determining to whom students would go for help if they felt the need for assistance. She surveyed 149 students in a diploma school of nursing, consisting of 61 freshmen, 54 juniors, and 34 seniors. The students were given a list of possible sources of help consisting of:

| | |
|---|---|
| Sister or brother | Friend |
| Teacher | Clergyman |
| Mother | Counselor |
| Father | Other |

It is important to note that the school did not have a counselor at the time the study was conducted, and had never had one. Students were asked to assume that one was available. They were then asked to rank the source of help in relation to the question, "To whom would you feel most free to go to with a problem?" It was assumed that there could be a difference of choice depending upon the nature of the problem, but students were asked to make decisions as to whom they would generally approach with their problems.

The results serve as an interesting reflection of student attitudes toward sources of assistance. This study can be analyzed in several ways.

Students seem to rely less on family resources as they gain experience and maturity; e.g. the reliance on siblings and parents drops from freshman to senior year. The reliance on faculty members also dropped, although they were never ranked high. Perhaps this is an indication of student fear of taking problems to faculty members who are also evaluating students. It is almost impossible to interpret the use of a counselor, since there was none in the school. It may be that student selection of a counselor was based on their previous relationship with a counselor in high school. This study would have been strengthened greatly by asking students to provide the reasons for their choices, yet it does serve at least to illustrate a simple attempt to look at current practice within a particular school regarding a particular service. This sort of study is important not only to gain a picture of student use of services, but also to aid in determining why students do or do not use a particular resource.

Ogston and Ogston (1970) were interested in approaching the problem of program evaluation from a somewhat different perspective. They used as a primary criterion of effectiveness the incidence of use of a counselor's time over a two-year period in a diploma school of nursing. In the fall of 1967 Calgary General Hospital School of Nursing set up a counseling service with three main functions: counseling the students, consulting with the faculty, and conducting research. A record was kept of the hours spent on each function during the first two years of the new service. It would seem that, from their results, both students and faculty increased their use of the counseling service over the two-year period. This may be due to a growth in acceptance of the service as it became known, and to the effectiveness of the services in the eyes of the consumers. Nevertheless these conclusions must be taken with caution, for insufficient data are provided for adequate support. Additional analysis is needed to give the results meaning. There is also a danger in this kind of study, for members of the counseling staff and faculty may become more concerned with numbers of hours spent than with quality of service. Even so, the results of such a study could still be a useful addition to a composite evaluation report.

Schindler (1971) studied guidance and counseling services in seven diploma schools of nursing in Ohio. She had three objectives in mind:
1. The types of guidance and counseling services available in seven diploma schools of nursing accredited by the NLN
2. Who provides the guidance and counseling services, and what are the qualifications and preparation of these individuals?
3. How do students in these schools feel regarding the effectiveness of the guidance and counseling services, and do they utilize the services available?

Three of the seven schools had a full-time guidance counseling program. Evaluation in the schools was done by a variety of methods:
1. A questionnaire to graduating students regarding all aspects of the school program
2. A questionnaire to graduates six months to a year after graduation regarding the total school program
3. Annual faculty evaluation of each aspect of the school.

Schindler sent a questionnaire to randomly selected faculty members and counselors in the seven schools. Twenty-seven of 30 questionnaires were returned. The faculty questionnaire was the following:

Questionnaire for faculty or other personnel doing counseling in a diploma school of nursing.

*Directions:*   The following questionnaire is related to your role in the counseling and guidance program in your school of nursing. Please do *not* sign your name.

1. What is your role in the total counseling program in your school of nursing?
2. What preparation have you had to fulfill your role? (e.g. courses, inservice meetings, workshops, etc.)
3. Do you feel qualified to carry out this role?
4. Do you feel that counselors should have teaching or administrative duties in addition to counseling responsibilities? Why or why not?
5. Any comments you wish to make regarding counseling services in diploma schools of nursing would be appreciated.

On the faculty questionnaire, the results are worth a brief analysis. On question 1, the majority of responses indicated that the respondents provided counseling services to students on either an assigned or voluntary basis. On question 2, slightly over half had received some form of preparation for a counseling role through workshops, in-service programs, or graduate work in counseling. On question 3, only a third of the respondents felt qualified to carry out a counseling role. Finally, on question 4, almost all felt that the counselor should be free of any teaching or administrative responsibilities.

In the second part of the study, a questionnaire was sent to randomly selected junior students in three of the seven schools of nursing. Of the 45 questionnaires distributed, 37 were returned. The questionnaire used was the following:

*Directions:*   The following questionnaire is a survey of the counseling and guidance services offered in your school of nursing. I would appreciate honest answers with any comments you wish to make. Names are *not* to be signed; this is to be anonymous.

*Questionnaire*

1. What do you think of when the terms "counseling" and "guidance" are used?
2. Did you understand the objectives and functions of the counseling program of your school when oriented?
   How did this compare with your high school counseling program?
3. What counseling service have you utilized in your school of nursing?
   a. Your specified counselor
   b. The instructor of a particular rotation
   c. Director of the school (or associate)
   d. Health nurse
   e. Any others— specify the title of the person

4. Could you have utilized more facilities than you did? If so, why didn't you?
5. Was any of your counseling done by your choice, or forced by someone?
6. Were you in any group counseling sessions? If so, was this as helpful to you as individual counseling?
7. Did you feel free to approach your counselor?
8. Did you feel that your counselor was qualified? What qualifications (personal and professional) do you expect a counselor to have?
9. Did you feel that your conversations were kept confidential?
10. Did you feel that any counseling you received was helpful? If so, how?
11. Can you suggest any improvements in the counseling program?

Again, the responses of the students provide an interesting commentary on program characteristics. A review of selected questions reveals the following answers: On question 2, 21 of the 37 students did not understand the objectives of the counseling program when oriented. This would indicate a definite need for revision of the orientation process to improve the awareness and understanding of the counseling services available to students. On question 4, 20 of the 37 felt that they could have utilized more facilities. When asked why they hadn't, 12 of the 20 gave reasons including lack of confidentiality, "shows a sign of weakness," "problem was not great enough," and "didn't want to hurt my assigned counselor." Again, this indicates the need for a reorientation to counseling.

Question 5 indicated that 26 of 37 received counseling at least partially on a forced basis. Only 8 of 37 students indicated any participation in group counseling, as reported in question 6. On question 7, 13 of 37 indicated that they did not feel free to approach their counselor. Twenty-two of 37 felt that their counselor was qualified, as reported in question 8. Finally, on question 9, only 18 of 37 felt that their conversations were kept confidential. This point is a vitally important one, revealing a real weakness in the programs.

The Schindler study is a useful one in suggesting problem areas. It would have been valuable to compare the student responses with those of faculty members and counselors from the same schools. Areas of disagreement could then be explored more thoroughly in terms of the implications for program revision and development.

## GENERAL OBSERVATIONS ON THE EVALUATION PROCESS

As mentioned earlier, the evaluation of the guidance, counseling, and student personnel program is a process rather than a single event occurring sporadically. Ideally, there are five stages in the evaluation process. In the first stage the faculty and administration develop a carefully thought-through philosophy of education as it applies to the particular school of nursing. This philosophy includes the broad goals of the school, along with the specific behavioral objectives to be reached in the process of educating student nurses. The philosophy, goals, and objectives are usually a composite of the stated purposes of the profession, the needs and expectations of society, and the creative thinking and beliefs of the faculty and administration within the school of nursing.

In the second stage the philosophy of the school is applied to the guidance, counseling, and student personnel program. This application depends on the way the faculty and administration view students and their needs. At times the philosophy may also be somewhat colored by the pressures and expectations of parents and the community at large. Once this is done, by means of a thorough and continuing process, the philosophy of the school and the goals and objectives of the student personnel program are translated to the students. Every possible means is used to implement the program in a way designed to maximize student growth and development, and to meet student and faculty needs and expectations.

Once the program is implemented, planning should immediately begin for the third stage, that of program evaluation. This should be done on a regular basis; as a general rule of thumb, systematic program evaluation should be conducted minimally every time the student body completely changes. For example, in AD programs, program evaluation should be done every third year; in diploma schools, every fourth year; and in baccalaureate programs, every fourth or fifth year, depending on the number of years the students are actually enrolled in the school of nursing. This minimal schedule is necessary because a program developed for today's students and with today's faculty may not be suitable for the new group once all the current group have graduated or left.

In the third stage, representatives from faculty, administration, and students as a combined committee should lay careful plans for a thorough self-study of the program. These plans should include procedures for surveying the faculty, students, graduates, withdrawals and terminations, and employers. The process of self-study may utilize an instrument such as the Rackham Inventory by itself, or with one or more questionnaires developed within the school. The plans should also provide for an ongoing process of data collection between evaluation periods; e.g. all students who leave the school prior to graduation for any reason are asked to complete an evaluation questionnaire along with an exit interview. The purposes of this comprehensive self-study should be carefully explained to all involved, including the confidentiality of information, and the way the data will be used.

After the collection of data in the third stage, the study committee is ready to move into the fourth stage, which is the analysis of results, the arrival at recommendations for change, and the plans for implementing wherever possible the recommendations reached. Unless careful plans are made to follow-up an evaluation study, the entire process represents almost a total waste of effort. The analysis of results should yield both short-range and long-range recommendations. Included should be a careful record of the evaluation process itself and recommendations for procedures to be followed for the next scheduled program evaluation.

The final stage is a necessary one, but one not used widely enough, i.e. the use of consultants to review the evaluation process, study results, and recommendations. Since our objective is to improve the guidance, counseling, and student personnel program, these consultants should be experts in these areas, particularly as they are conducted in schools of nursing. We are referring here to a team of consultants selected by the committee, with whom there is mutual confidence and trust. The consultant committee would be asked to review all phases of the self-study and to react to its validity and reliability. A good consultant committee can greatly increase the value to be gained from a self-study.

In summary, evaluation involves accountability; i.e. every phase of the program must be made regularly accountable for its successes and failures in order to justify its existence. Program evaluation is vitally necessary if the decision-making process is to move beyond the realm of personal opinion. It will inevitably involve risk, both in the study process itself and in the implementation of change from the status quo. Thus a good evaluation is usually the product of a secure study committee functioning in an open and democratic school of nursing with mutual trust and cooperation.

# BIBLIOGRAPHY

## Part 3

Adams, Jerry, and Klein, Lilyan R.: Students in Nursing School: Considerations in Assessing Personality Characteristics. *Nursing Research,* Vol. 19, No. 4, 1970, pp. 362–366.

Aldag, Jean C.: Occupational and Nonoccupational Interest Characteristics of Men Nurses. *Nursing Research,* Vol. 19, No. 6, 1970, pp. 529–533.

Armacost, Peter H.: Student Personnel Administration Policies; in Asa A. Knowles (Ed.): *Handbook of College and University Administration—Academic Volume.* New York, McGraw-Hill Book Co., Inc., 1970.

Bailey, June T., and Claus, Karen E.: Comparative Analysis of the Personality Structure of Nursing Students. *Nursing Research,* Vol. 18, No. 4, 1969, pp. 320–326.

Baldwin, Jean P., Mowbray, Jean K., and Taylor, Jr., Raymond G.: Factors Influencing Performance on State Board Test Pool Examination. *Nursing Research,* Vol. 17, No. 2, 1968, p. 170.

Berg, Irwin August: Study of Success and Failure Among Student Nurses. *Journal of Applied Psychology,* Vol. 31, August, 1947, pp. 389–396.

Bernfeld, Benjamin: MMPI Variables in the Prediction of Attrition of Students of Nursing in a Hospital School Program. Unpublished Doctoral Dissertation, New York University, 1967.

Black, Hillel: *They Shall Not Pass.* New York, Morrow, 1963.

Bloland, Paul A.: Student Activities; in Asa A. Knowles (Ed.): *Handbook of College and University Administration—Academic Volume.* New York, McGraw-Hill Book Company, Inc., 1970.

Bowers, William J., and Salem, Richard G.: Disciplinary Administration—Traditional and New; in Asa A. Knowles (Ed.): *Handbook of College and University Administration—Academic Volume.* New York, McGraw-Hill Book Company, Inc., 1970.

Brandt, Edna Mae, Hastie, Bettinas, and Schumann, Dolores: Predicting Success on State Board Examinations. *Nursing Research,* Vol. 15, No. 1, Winter, 1966, pp. 62–69.

Brown, Dirck W.: Interpreting the College Student to Prospective Employers, Government Agencies, and Graduate Schools. *Personnel & Guidance Journal,* Vol. 39, No. 7, 1961, pp. 576–582.

Brown, William F., and Holtzman, Wayne H.: *Survey of Study Habits and Attitudes.* New York, The Psychological Corporation, 1967.

Burgess, Michall, and Duffey, Margery: The Prediction of Success in a Collegiate Program of Nursing. *Nursing Research,* Vol. 18, No. 1, 1969, pp. 69–72.

Committee on Credit by Examination, University of Arizona, College of Nursing: Let's Examine—The Challenge Examination for the Registered Nurse Student. *Nursing Outlook,* Vol. 17, No. 4, 1969, p. 48.

Coulter, Pearl Parson: This I Believe—About Recruitment in an Age of Change. *Nursing Outlook,* Vol. 14, No. 4, 1966, pp. 31–33.

Crider, Blake: A School of Nursing Selection Program. *Journal of Applied Psychology,* Vol. 27, October, 1943, pp. 452–457.

*Criteria for the Evaluation of Diploma Programs in Nursing.* New York, National League for Nursing, 1969.

Deegan, William L., Drexel, Karl O., Collins, John T., and Kearney, Dorothy L.: Student Participation in Governance. *Junior College Journal,* Vol. 41, No. 3, November, 1970, pp. 15–22.

DeFrank, Sister Joseph Leo: RIPS: A Remedial Instruction Program. *Nursing Outlook,* Vol. 19, No. 3, 1971, pp. 180–181.

Derian, Al: Cost and Utility in Reduction of Scholastic Attrition in Associate Degree Programs in Nursing. *College Journal,* 1962.

DeLourdes, Sister M., and Ary, Donald E.: Let's Examine—PGN, HSR and Licensure Examination Results. *Nursing Outlook,* Vol. 15, No. 11, 1967, p. 66.

Dorffeld, Mildred E., Ray, Thomas S., and Baumberger, Theodore S.: A Study of Selection Criteria for Nursing School Applicants. *Nursing Research,* Vol. 7, June, 1958.

Educational Testing Service, Cooperative Test Division: *Cooperative English Tests.* Princeton, N.J., Berkeley, Calif., 1961.

*Edwards Personal Preference Schedule.* New York, The Psychological Corporation, 1954.

Fillmore, Genevieve: When You Are Asked About Nursing. *American Journal of Nursing,* Vol. 63, No. 8, 1963, pp. 74–76.

Flanagan, John C., Gosnell, Doris, and Fivars, Grace: Evaluating Student Performance. *American Journal of Nursing,* Vol. 63, No. 11, November, 1963, pp. 96–99.

Fleming, Robben W., and others: *Statement on Student-Faculty-Administrative Relationships.* National Association of State Universities and Land Grant Colleges, November, 1969.

Fordyce, Joseph W.: Creating a Good Climate; in Seldon Menefee and Jack Orcult (Eds.): *Focus on Action.* Washington, D.C., American Association of Junior Colleges, May, 1969.

Franckleton, Dorothy, and Faville, Katharine: Opportunities in Nursing for Disadvantaged Youth. *Nursing Outlook,* Vol. 14, No. 4, 1966, pp. 26–28.

French, Joseph L.: A Predictive Test Battery. *Nursing Research,* Vol. 10, No. 2, Spring, 1961.

Garrett, Wiley S.: Prediction of Academic Success in a School of Nursing. *Personnel and Guidance Journal,* Vol. 38, 1960, pp. 500–503.

Gerstein, Alvin I.: Development of a Selection Program for Nursing Candidates. *Nursing Research,* Vol. 14, No. 3, Summer, 1965, pp. 254–257.

Girona, Ricardo: The Semantic Differential as a Tool in Predicting the Potential Effectiveness of Student Nurses. Unpublished Doctoral Dissertation, University of Florida, 1969.

Goza, John Thomas: An Investigation of the Academic Potential, Academic Achievement and Personality of Participants in an Associate Degree Nursing Program. Unpublished Doctoral Dissertation, East Texas State University, 1970.

Green, Edith Josephine: The Relationship of Self-Actualization to Achievement in Nursing. Unpublished Doctoral Dissertation, Indiana University, 1967.

Gross, Martin L.: *The Brain Watchers.* New York, Random House, 1962.

Grundeman, Barbara J., and Staff of NLN Test Services: Let's Examine—Prediction of Attrition in a Diploma Program. *Nursing Outlook,* Vol. 15, No. 5, 1967, p. 66.

Gunter, Laurie M.: The Developing Nursing Student. Part I. A Study of Self-Actualizing Values. *Nursing Research,* Vol. 18, No. 1, 1969, pp. 60–64.

Hage, Robert S.: A Revision of the Rackham Student Personnel Services Inventory. Unpublished Doctoral Dissertation, State University of Iowa, Iowa City, Iowa, 1957.

Harvey, Lillian H.: Educational Problems of Minority Group Nurses. *Nursing Outlook,* Vol. 18, No. 9, 1970, pp. 48–50.

Hedlund, Dalvna E.: Preparation for Student Personnel: Implications of Humanistic Education. *Journal of College Student Personnel,* Vol. 12, No. 5, September, 1971, pp. 324–328.

Heidgerken, Loretta: Nursing as a Career: Is It Relevant? *American Journal of Nursing,* Vol. 69, No. 6, June, 1969, pp. 1217–1222.

Henke, Sister Grace: Project Tap—A Tutorial Program. *American Journal of Nursing*, Vol. 71, No. 5, May, 1971, pp. 978–981.

Hill, Lorraine Loy, Taylor, Calvin, and Stacy, Jane E.: Attrition in Nursing Schools and Job Turnover in Professional Nursing. *Nursing Outlook*, Vol. 11, No. 9, 1963, pp. 666–669.

Hoffman, Banesh: *The Tyranny of Testing.* New York, Crowell-Collier, 1962.

Johnson, Nancy: Recruitment of Minority Groups—A Priority for NSNA. *Nursing Outlook*, Vol. 14, No. 4, 1966, pp. 29–30.

Johnson, Richard W., and Leonard, Louise C.: Psychological Test Characteristics and Performance of Nursing Students. *Nursing Research*, Vol. 19, No. 2, 1970, pp. 147–150.

Kaback, Goldie Ruth: *Guidance and Counseling Perspectives for Hospital Schools of Nursing.* New York, National League for Nursing, 1958.

Katzell, Mildred E.: Let's Examine—Student Expectation and Dropouts from Schools of Nursing. *Nursing Outlook*, Vol. 15, No. 7, 1967, p. 63.

Katzell, Mildred E.: Expectations and Dropouts in Schools of Nursing. *Journal of Applied Psychology*, Vol. 52, No. 2, 1968, pp. 154–157.

Katzell, Mildred, E.: Upward Mobility in Nursing. *Nursing Outlook*, Vol. 18, No. 9, 1970, pp. 36–39.

Kennedy, Janet: A Workshop for High School Counselors. *Nursing Outlook*, Vol. 9, No. 8, 1961, p. 493.

Kirk, Barbara, Goodstein, Leonard, and Cummings, Rogers: The Strong Vocational Interest Blank and Collegiate Nursing Education. *Personnel and Guidance Journal*, Vol. 40, 1961, pp. 160–163.

Klahn, James Edward: An Analysis of Selected Factors and Success of First Year Student Nurses. Unpublished Doctoral Dissertation, Washington State University, 1966.

Klahn, James Edward: Self Concept and Change Seeking Need of First Year Student Nurses. *Journal of Nursing Education*, Vol. 8, No. 2, 1969, pp. 11–16.

Klassen, Kathryn L., and White, Joanne: Health Career Day at Dodge City. *Nursing Outlook*, Vol. 19, No. 3, 1971, pp. 168–169.

Klemer, Margaret: Counselors' Image of the Basic Nursing Student. *Nursing Outlook*, Vol. 12, No. 10, 1964.

Knowles, Lois N.: Attracting Nurses for Tomorrow. *American Journal of Nursing*, Vol. 61, No. 9, September, 1961, pp. 80–82.

Kovacs, Alberta Rose: Predicting Success in Three Selected Collegiate Schools of Nursing. Unpublished Doctoral Dissertation, Columbia University, 1968.

Kovacs, Alberta Rose: Uniform Minimum Admission Standards. *Nursing Outlook*, Vol. 18, No. 10, 1970, pp. 54–56.

Langheim, Isidore A.: The Prediction of Poor Achievement on Three Year Nurses Training from Deviation Scores and Personality Test. Unpublished Master's Thesis, John Carroll University, 1966.

Ledbetter, Peggy Jean: An Analysis of the Performance of Graduates of a Selected Baccalaureate Program in Nursing with Regard to Selected Standardized Examinations. Unpublished Doctoral Dissertation, University of Alabama, 1968.

Leonetti, Ann Marie: The Status of Guidance Services for Potential Nurse Candidates in Selected Senior High Schools. *Journal of Nursing Education*, Vol. 4, No. 3, 1965, pp. 9–13.

Lindstrom, May Rizpah: Student Survival in a Collegiate Basic Nursing Program. Unpublished Doctoral Dissertation, Stanford University, 1961.

Litherland, Ronald Lee: The Iowa Tests of Educational Development as a Predictor of Academic Success in Iowa Schools of Professional Nursing. Unpublished Doctoral Dissertation, University of Iowa, 1966.

Litwack, Lawrence, Getson, Russell, and Saltzman, Glenn: *Research in Counseling.* Itasca, Ill., F. E. Peacock, 1968.

Ludwig, Helen G.: Study of Preferences for Confidants of Students in a School of Nursing. Unpublished term paper, Kent State University, 1968.

Lukens, Lois Graham: The Nurse Stereotype Must Go. *Vocational Guidance Quarterly*, Vol. 13, No. 2, 1964–1965, pp. 95–99.

McKaig, Richard: A Proposed Statement for ACPA Regarding Student Participation in the Governance of Institutions of Higher Learning. *Journal of College Student Personnel*, Vol. 12, No. 5, September, 1971, pp. 388–389.

Malkin, Evelyn: Direction or Dilemma for RNs in Baccalaureate Education. *Nursing Outlook*, Vol. 14, No. 5, 1966, pp. 36–39.

Mancott, Anatole: Let's Examine—Prediction of Performance in Chemistry. *Nursing Outlook,* Vol. 17, No. 11, 1969, p. 55.

Mancott, Anatole: Let's Examine—Prediction of Performance in Chemistry. II. *Nursing Outlook,* Vol. 18, No. 11, 1970, p. 57.

Meadow, Lloyd, and Edelson, Ruth E.: Age and Marital Status. *Nursing Outlook,* Vol. 11, No. 4, 1963, p. 289.

Meluskey, Mary M.: Student Relations. Notes from 12th Annual Workshop for Faculties of Schools of Nursing, Penn State University, June, 1971.

Mereness, Dorothy: Freedom and Responsibility for Nursing Students. *American Journal of Nursing,* Vol. 67, No. 1, January, 1967, pp. 69–71.

Metz, Edith Martin: Development of a Standardized Test of Cognitive Aspects of Efficient Body Movement for Technical and Professional Nursing Students. Unpublished Doctoral Dissertation, University of Washington, 1964.

Metzler, John H.: Evaluating Counseling and Guidance Programs. *Vocational Guidance Quarterly,* Vol. 12, No. 4, 1964, pp. 285–289.

Michael, William B., Haney, Russell, and Brown, Stephen W.: The Predictive Validity of a Battery of Diversified Measures Related to Success in Student Nursing. *Educational & Psychological Measurement,* Vol. 25, No. 2, June, 1965, p. 579–583.

Miller, Carol L., and others: The Prediction of State Board Examinations Scores of Graduates of an Associate Degree Program. *Nursing Research,* Vol. 17, No. 6, 1968, pp. 555–558.

Mowbray, Jean K., and Taylor, Raymond G.: Validity of Interest Inventories for the Prediction of Success in Schools of Nursing. *Nursing Research,* Vol. 16, 1967, pp. 78–81.

Muhlenkamp, Ann F.: Let's Examine—Prediction of State Board Scores in a Baccalaureate Program. *Nursing Outlook,* Vol. 19, No. 1, 1971, p. 57.

Muldrow, Catherine: Now It's Students of Nursing. *American Journal of Nursing,* Vol. 69, No. 6, June, 1969, pp. 1252–1253.

Munday, Leo., and Hoyt, Donald P.: Predicting Academic Success for Nursing Students. *Nursing Research,* Vol. 14, No. 4, Fall, 1965, pp. 341–344.

O'Banion, Terry, Thurston, Alice, and Gulden, James: Student Personnel Work: An Emerging Model. *Junior College Journal,* Vol. 41, No. 3, November, 1970, pp. 6–14.

Ogston, Donald G., and Ogston, Karen M.: Counseling Students in a Hospital School of Nursing. *The Canadian Nurse,* Vol. 66, April, 1970, pp. 52–53.

Osgood, Gretchen A.: Dimensions of Involvement. *Nursing Outlook,* Vol. 17, No. 19, 1969.

Papcam, Ida D.: Let's Examine—Results of Achievement Tests and State Board Tests in an Associate Degree Program. *Nursing Outlook,* Vol. 19, No. 5, 1971, p. 341.

Parker, Cherry: Recruiting at High School "College Days." *Nursing Outlook,* Vol. 12, No. 12, 1964, pp. 38–39.

Peterson, Carol Jean Willts: Secondary School Counselors' and Nurse Educators' Perceptions of Trends in Nursing Education and Images of Nursing. Unpublished Doctoral Dissertation, University of Minnesota, 1969.

Rackham, Eric N.: The Determination of Criteria for the Evaluation of Student Personnel Services in Institutions of Higher Learning. Unpublished Doctoral Dissertation, University of Michigan, 1951.

Reekie, Elagrace: Personality Factors and Biographical Characteristics Associated with Criterion Behaviors of Success in Professional Nursing. Unpublished Doctoral Dissertation, University of Washington, 1970.

Richter, Lucretia: Project Late Start. *Nursing Outlook,* Vol. 17, No. 3, 1969, pp. 35–36.

Riker, Harold C.: Housing; in Asa S. Knowles (Ed.); *Handbook of College and University Administration.* New York, McGraw-Hill Book Company, Inc., 1970.

Rotter, Julian B.: *Incomplete Sentences Blank Adult Form.* New York, Psychological Corporation, 1950.

Rottkamp, Barbara C.: Attrition Rates in Basic Baccalaureate Programs. *Nursing Outlook,* Vol. 16 No. 6, 1969, pp. 44–47.

Ryder, Cecil A., Jr., and Wilson, Fay O.: The Power of Positive Student Action. *Nursing Outlook,* Vol. 17, No. 3, March, 1969.

Scheinfeldt, Jean, and Palmer, Sarena R.: Expansion: New Youth for Nursing. *American Journal of Nursing,* Vol. 70, No. 8, August, 1970, pp. 1713–1717.

Schindler, Janet: A Comparison of the Counseling and Guidance Program in Selected Diploma Schools of Nursing. Ind. Inv. paper, Kent State University, 1971.

Schulz, Esther D.: Personality Traits of Nursing Students and Faculty Concepts of Desirable

Traits: A Longitudinal Comparative Study. *Nursing Research,* Vol. 14, No. 3, Summer, 1965, pp. 261–264.

Seegars, James E., Rogers, George W., and Denny, Charlotte: Leary Interpersonal Diagnosis of Freshman Nursing Students. *Nursing Outlook,* Vol. 11, No. 9, 1963, p. 670.

Staff of NLN Measurement and Evaluation Services: Let's Examine—An Annotated Bibliography on Challenge Examinations. *Nursing Outlook,* Vol. 17, No. 10, 1969, pp. 60–61.

Staff of NLN Measurement and Evaluation Services: Let's Examine—The Selection of Proficiency Examination. *Nursing Outlook,* Vol. 17, No. 12, 1969, p. 36.

Staff of NLN Measurement and Evaluation Services: Let's Examine—The Validity of NLN Pre-Nursing and Guidance Examination. *Nursing Outlook,* Vol. 18, No. 3, March, 1970, p. 56.

Staff of NLN Measurement and Evaluation Service: Let's Examine—PNG Performance and Performance in a School of Nursing. *Nursing Outlook,* Vol. 18, No. 4, 1970, p. 55.

Staff of NLN Measurement and Evaluation Service: Let's Examine—PNG Performance and Academic Ratings. *Nursing Outlook,* Vol. 18, No. 5, 1970, p. 66.

Staff of NLN Measurement and Evaluation Service: Let's Examine—Performance on PNG and State Board Examination. *Nursing Outlook,* Vol. 18, No. 6, 1970, p. 62–63.

Staff of NLN Measurement and Evaluation Services: Let's Examine—PNG Performance and Race. *Nursing Outlook,* Vol. 18, No. 7, 1970, p. 41.

Staff of NLN Measurement and Evaluation Service: Let's Examine—The Relationship of State Board and Achievement Test Performance. *Nursing Outlook,* Vol. 18, No. 8, 1970, p. 61.

Staff of NLN Measurement and Evaluation Service: Let's Examine—The Revised Pre-Nursing and Guidance Examination. *Nursing Outlook,* Vol. 19, No. 8, August, 1971, p. 537.

Staff of NLN Test Services: Let's Examine—The NLN Course End and Comprehensive Achievement Tests. *Nursing Outlook,* Vol. 9, No. 7, 1961, p. 431.

Staff of NLN Test Services: Let's Examine—Standardized Tests—Reflections or Promoters of Change. *Nursing Outlook,* Vol. 10, No. 8, 1962, p. 532.

Staff of NLN Test Services: Let's Examine—Differences of Test Scores of Students in Diploma and Degree Programs. *Nursing Outlook,* Vol. 10, No. 9, 1962, p. 617.

Staff of NLN Test Service: Let's Examine—Safety and Effectiveness of Practice. *Nursing Outlook,* Vol. 10, No. 10, 1962, p. 679.

Staff of NLN Test Services: Let's Examine—The Content of NLN Entrance Examinations. *Nursing Outlook,* Vol. 11, No. 2, Feb., 1963, p. 137.

Staff of NLN Test Services: Composite Scores on Selection Tests. *Nursing Outlook,* Vol. 11, No. 9, 1963, p. 672.

Staff of NLN Test Services: Let's Examine—Why One Licensure Examination. *Nursing Outlook,* Vol. 11, No. 10, 1963, p. 749.

Staff of NLN Test Services: Let's Examine—The Testing of Application of Facts and Principles. *Nursing Outlook,* Vol. 11, No. 12, 1963, p. 908.

Staff of NLN Test Services: The History of Plans for Licensure Tests in Professional Nursing. *Nursing Outlook,* Vol. 12, No. 8, 1964, p. 55.

Staff of NLN Test Services: Let's Examine—The Graduate Nurse Examination, Past and Future. *Nursing Outlook,* Vol. 13, No. 2, 1965, p. 39.

Staff of NLN Test Services: Let's Examine—Separate Licensure Examinations for Diploma and Degree Program Graduates. *Nursing Outlook,* Vol. 13, No. 7, 1965, p. 51.

Staff of NLN Test Services: Let's Examine—Tides of Change in Psychiatric Nursing. *Nursing Outlook,* Vol. 13, No. 11, 1965, p. 60.

Staff of NLN Test Services: Let's Examine—Development of a National League for Nursing Standardized Achievement Test. *Nursing Outlook,* Vol. 14, No. 3, 1966, p. 65.

Staff of NLN Test Services: Let's Examine—Preparing Students to Take NLN Achievement Tests. *Nursing Outlook,* Vol. 14, No. 12, 1966, p. 59.

Staff of NLN Test Services: Let's Examine—Multiple Regression and Multiple Cutoffs. *Nursing Outlook,* Vol. 15, No. 10, 1967, p. 61.

Staff of NLN Test Services: *Toward Excellence in Nursing Education—A Guide for Diploma School Improvement.* New York, National League for Nursing, 1971.

Student Nurses Association of Illinois: Student Bill of Rights. Unpublished document, 1969.

Tannenbaum, Robert, and Davis, Sheldon A.: Values, Man, and Organizations; in William B. Eddy and others (Eds.); *Behavioral Science and the Manager's Role.* Washington, D.C., NTL Institute for Applied Behavioral Science, 1969.

Taylor, C. W., and others: *Selection and Recruitment of Nurses and Nursing Students: A Review of Research Studies and Practices.* Salt Lake City, University of Utah Press, 1966.

Thomas, Mary Ann: Admissions Criteria as a Prediction of Success. Unpublished Master's Thesis, Kent State University, 1967.

Thurston, John, Brunclik, Helen, and Finn, Pat: The Fall out Problem in Nursing Education. *Nursing Forum,* Vol. 1, 1962, pp. 90–97.

Thurston, John R., and Brunclik, Helen L.: The Relationship of Personality to Achievement in Nursing Education. *Nursing Research,* Vol. 14, No. 2, Spring, 1965, pp. 203–209.

Vickery, Myra S.: Nightingales from Yellow Birds. *American Journal of Nursing,* Vol. 70, No. 10, October, 1970, pp. 2158–2159.

Wilson, Christopher: The Effects of Cloisterization on Students of Nursing. *American Journal of Nursing,* Vol. 70, No. 8, August, 1970, pp. 1726–1729.

Yates, Judith A.: Breakthrough in Minnesota. *American Journal of Nursing,* Vol. 70, No. 3, March, 1970, pp. 563–565.

# *Appendix:*

# *Joint Statement on Rights and Freedoms of Students*

In June, 1967, a joint committee, comprised of representatives from the American Association of University Professors, U.S. National Student Association, Association of American Colleges, National Association of Student Personnel Administrators, and National Association of Women Deans and Counselors, met in Washington, D.C., and drafted the following *Joint Statement on Rights and Freedoms of Students.* Since its formulation, the Joint Statement has been endorsed by each of its five national sponsors, as well as by a number of other professional bodies.

## PREAMBLE

Academic institutions exist for the transmission of knowledge, the pursuit of truth, the development of students, and the general well-being of society. Free inquiry and free expression are indispensable to the attainment of these goals. As members of the academic community, students should be encouraged to develop the capacity for critical judgment and to engage in a sustained and independent search for truth. Institutional procedures for achieving these purposes may vary from campus to campus, but the minimal standards of academic freedom of students outlined below are essential to any community of scholars.

Freedom to teach and freedom to learn are inseparable facets of academic freedom. The freedom to learn depends upon appropriate opportunities and conditions in the classroom, on the campus, and in the larger community. Students should exercise their freedom with responsibility.

The responsibility to secure and to respect general conditions conducive to the freedom to learn is shared by all members of the academic community. Each college and university has a duty to develop policies and procedures which provide and safeguard this freedom. Such policies and procedures should be developed at each institution within the framework of general standards and with the broadest possible participation of the members of the academic community. The purpose of this statement is to enumerate the essential provisions for student freedom to learn.

## I. FREEDOM OF ACCESS TO HIGHER EDUCATION

The admissions policies of each college and university are a matter of institutional choice provided that each college and university makes clear the characteristics and expectations of students which it considers relevant to success in the institution's program. While church-related institutions may give admission preference to students of their own persuasion, such a preference should be clearly and publicly stated. Under no circumstances should a student be barred from admission to a particular institution on the basis of race. Thus, within the limits of its facilities, each college and university should be open to all students who are qualified according to its admission standards. The facilities and services of a college should be open to all of its enrolled students, and institutions should use their

234

influence to secure equal access for all students to public facilities in the local community.

## II. IN THE CLASSROOM

The professor in the classroom and in conference should encourage free discussion, inquiry, and expression. Student performance should be evaluated solely on an academic basis, not on opinions or conduct in matters unrelated to academic standards.

### A. Protection of Freedom of Expression

Students should be free to take reasoned exception to the data or views offered in any course of study and to reserve judgment about matters of opinion, but they are responsible for learning the content of any course of study for which they are enrolled.

### B. Protection Against Improper Academic Evaluation

Students should have protection through orderly procedures against prejudiced or capricious academic evaluation. At the same time, they are responsible for maintaining standards of academic performance established for each course in which they are enrolled.

### C. Protection Against Improper Disclosure

Information about student views, beliefs, and political associations which professors acquire in the course of their work as instructors, advisers, and counselors should be considered confidential. Protection against improper disclosure is a serious professional obligation. Judgments of ability and character may be provided under appropriate circumstances, normally with the knowledge or consent of the student.

## III. STUDENT RECORDS

Institutions should have a carefully considered policy as to the information which should be part of a student's permanent educational record and as to the conditions of its disclosure. To minimize the risk of improper disclosure, academic and disciplinary records should be separate, and the conditions of access to each should be set forth in an explicit policy statement. Transcripts of academic records should contain only information about academic status. Information from disciplinary or counseling files should not be available to unauthorized persons on campus, or to any person off campus without the express consent of the student involved except under legal compulsion or in cases where the safety of persons or property is involved. No records should be kept which reflect the political activities or beliefs of students. Provisions should also be made for periodic routine destruction of noncurrent disciplinary records. Administrative staff and faculty members should respect confidential information about students which they acquire in the course of their work.

## IV. STUDENT AFFAIRS

In student affairs, certain standards must be maintained if the freedom of students is to be preserved.

### A. Freedom of Association

Students bring to the campus a variety of interests previously acquired and develop many new interests as members of the academic community. They should be free to organize and join associations to promote their common interests.

1. The membership, policies, and actions of a student organization usually will be determined by vote of only those persons who hold bona fide membership in the college or university community.

2. Affiliation with an extramural organization should not of itself disqualify a student organization from institutional recognition.

3. If campus advisers are required, each organization should be free to choose its own adviser, and institutional recognition should not be withheld or withdrawn solely because of the inability of a student organization to secure an adviser. Campus advisers may advise organizations in the exercise of responsibility, but they should not have the authority to control the policy of such organizations.

4. Student organizations may be required to submit a statement of purpose, criteria for membership, rules of procedures, and a current list of officers. They should not be required to submit a membership list as a condition of institutional recognition.

5. Campus organizations, including those affiliated with an extramural organization, should be open to all students without respect to race, creed, or national origin, except for religious qualifications which may be required by organizations whose aims are primarily sectarian.

### B. Freedom of Inquiry and Expression

1. Students and student organizations should be free to examine and discuss all questions of interest to them, and to express opinions publicly and privately. They should always be free to support causes by orderly means which do not disrupt the regular and essential operation of the institution. At the same time, it should be made clear to the academic and the larger community that in their public expressions or demonstrations students or student organizations speak only for themselves.

2. Students should be allowed to invite and to hear any person of their own choosing. Those routine procedures required by an institution before a guest speaker is invited to appear on campus should be designed only to insure that there is orderly scheduling of facilities and adequate preparation for the event, and that the occasion is conducted in a manner appropriate to an academic community. The institutional control of campus facilities should not be used as a device of censorship. It should be made clear to the academic and large community that sponsor-

---

*From the A.A.U.P. Bulletin, Vol. 54, Summer, 1968. Reprinted with permission.

ship of guest speakers does not necessarily imply approval or endorsement of the views expressed, either by the sponsoring group or the institution.

## C. Student Participation in Institutional Government

As constituents of the academic community, students should be free, individually and collectively, to express their views on issues of institutional policy and on matters of general interest to the student body. The student body should have clearly defined means to participate in the formulation and application of institutional policy affecting academic and student affairs. The role of the student government and both its general and specific responsibilities should be made explicit, and the actions of the student government within the areas of its jurisdiction should be reviewed only through orderly and prescribed procedures.

## D. Student Publications

Student publications and the student press are a valuable aid in establishing and maintaining an atmosphere of free and responsible discussion and of intellectual exploration on the campus. They are a means of bringing student concerns to the attention of the faculty and the institutional authorities and of formulating student opinion on various issues on the campus and in the world at large.

Whenever possible the student newspaper should be an independent corporation financially and legally separate from the university. Where financial and legal autonomy is not possible, the institution, as the publisher of student publications, may have to bear the legal responsibility for the contents of the publications. In the delegation of editorial responsibility to students the institution must provide sufficient editorial freedom and financial autonomy for the student publications to maintain their integrity of purpose as vehicles for free inquiry and free expression in an academic community.

Institutional authorities, in consultation with students and faculty, have a responsibility to provide written clarification of the role of the student publications, the standards to be used in their evaluation, and the limitations on external control of their operation. At the same time, the editorial freedom of student editors and managers entails corollary responsibilities to be governed by the canons of responsible journalism, such as the avoidance of libel, indecency, undocumented allegations, attacks on personal integrity, and the techniques of harassment and innuendo. As safeguards for the editorial freedom of student publications the following provisions are necessary.

1. The student press should be free of censorship and advance approval of copy, and its editors and managers should be free to develop their own editorial policies and news coverage.

2. Editors and managers of student publications should be protected from arbitrary suspension and removal because of student, faculty, administrative, or public disapproval of editorial policy or content. Only for proper and stated causes should editors and managers be subject to removal and then by orderly and prescribed procedures. The agency responsible for the appointment of editors and managers should be the agency responsible for their removal.

3. All university published and financed student publications should explicitly state on the editorial page that the opinions there expressed are not necessarily those of the college, university, or student body.

## V. OFF-CAMPUS FREEDOM OF STUDENTS

### A. *Exercise of Rights of Citizenship*

College and university students are both citizens and members of the academic community. As citizens, students should enjoy the same freedom of speech, peaceful assembly, and right of petition that other citizens enjoy and, as members of the academic community, they are subject to the obligations which accrue to them by virtue of this membership. Faculty members and administrative officials should insure that institutional powers are not employed to inhibit such intellectual and personal development of students as is often promoted by their exercise of the rights of citizenship both on and off campus.

### B. *Institutional Authority and Civil Penalties*

Activities of students may upon occasion result in violation of law. In such cases, institutional officials should be prepared to apprise students of sources of legal counsel and may offer other assistance. Students who violate the law may incur penalties prescribed by civil authorities, but institutional authority should never be used merely to duplicate the function of general laws. Only where the institution's interests as an academic community are distinct and clearly involved should the special authority of the institution be asserted. The student who incidentally violates institutional regulations in the course of his off-campus activity, such as those relating to class attendance, should be subject to no greater penalty than would normally be imposed. Institutional action should be independent of community pressure.

## VI. PROCEDURAL STANDARDS IN DISCIPLINARY PROCEEDINGS

In developing responsible student conduct, disciplinary proceedings play a role substantially secondary to example, counseling, guidance, and admonition. At the same time, educational institutions have a duty and the corollary disciplinary powers to protect their educational purpose through the setting of standards of scholarship and conduct for the students who attend them and through the regulation of the use of institutional facilities. In the exceptional circumstances when the preferred means fail to resolve problems of student conduct, proper procedural safeguards should be observed to protect the student from the unfair imposition of serious penalties.

The administration of discipline should guarantee procedural fairness to an accused student. Practices in disciplinary cases may vary in formality with the gravity of the offense and the sanctions which may be applied. They should also take into account the presence or absence of an honor code, and the degree to which the institutional officials have direct acquaintance with student life in general and with the involved student and the circumstances of the case in particular. The jurisdictions of faculty or student judicial bodies, the disciplinary responsibilities of institutional officials and the regular disciplinary procedures, including the student's right to appeal a decision, should be clearly formulated and communicated in advance. Minor penalties may be assessed informally under prescribed procedures.

In all situations, procedural fair play requires that the student be informed of the nature of the charges against him, that he be given a fair opportunity to refute them, that the institution not be arbitrary in its actions, and that there be provision for appeal of a decision. The following are recommended as proper safeguards in such proceedings when there are no honor codes offering comparable guarantees.

## A. Standards of Conduct Expected of Students

The institution has an obligation to clarify those standards of behavior which it considers essential to its educational mission and its community life. These general behavioral expectations and the resultant specific regulations should represent a reasonable regulation of student conduct, but the student should be as free as possible from imposed limitations that have no direct relevance to his education. Offenses should be as clearly defined as possible and interpreted in a manner consistent with the aforementioned principles of relevancy and reasonableness. Disciplinary proceedings should be instituted only for violations of standards of conduct formulated with significant student participation and published in advance through such means as a student handbook or a generally available body of institutional regulations.

## B. Investigation of Student Conduct

1. Except under extreme emergency circumstances, premises occupied by students and the personal possessions of students should not be searched unless appropriate authorization has been obtained. For premises such as residence halls controlled by the institution, an appropriate and responsible authority should be designated to whom application should be made before a search is conducted. The application should specify the reasons for the search and the objects or information sought. The student should be present, if possible, during the search. For premises not controlled by the institution, the ordinary requirements for lawful search should be followed.

2. Students detected or arrested in the course of serious violations of institutional regulations, or infractions of ordinary law, should be informed of their rights. No form of harassment should be used by institutional representatives to coerce admissions of guilt or information about conduct of other suspected persons.

## C. Status of Student Pending Final Action

Pending action on the charges, the status of a student should not be altered, or his right to be present on the campus and to attend classes suspended, except for reasons relating to the safety and well-being of students, faculty, or university property.

## D. Hearing Committee Procedures

When the misconduct may result in serious penalties and if the student questions the fairness of disciplinary action taken against him, he should be granted, on request, the privilege of a hearing before a regularly constituted hearing committee.

The following suggested hearing committee procedures satisfy the requirements of procedural due process in situations requiring a high degree of formality.

1. The hearing committee should include faculty members or students, or, if regularly included or requested by the accused, both faculty and student members. No member of the hearing committee who is otherwise interested in the particular case should sit in judgment during the proceeding.

2. The student should be informed, in writing, of the reasons for the proposed disciplinary action with sufficient particularity, and in sufficient time, to insure opportunity to prepare for the hearing.

3. The student appearing before the hearing committee should have the right to be assisted in his defense by an adviser of his choice.

4. The burden of proof should rest upon the officials bringing the charge.

5. The student should be given an opportunity to testify and to present evidence and witnesses. He should have an opportunity to hear and question adverse witnesses. In no case should the committee consider statements against him unless he has been advised of their content and of the names of those who made them and unless he has been given an opportunity to rebut unfavorable inferences which might otherwise be drawn.

6. All matters upon which the decision may be based must be introduced into evidence at the proceeding before the hearing committee. The decision should be based solely upon such matters. Improperly acquired evidence should not be admitted.

7. In the absence of a transcript, there should be both a digest and a verbatim record, such as a tape recording, of the hearing.

8. The decision of the hearing committee should be final, subject only to the student's right of appeal to the president or ultimately to the governing board of the institution.

# Index

Abortion, 60
Absences, classroom, 11
Admission(s), and records, 182–192
  criteria for, 182
Advising, 5
Advisor, faculty, 26
Alcohol, abuse of, 49
Attendance irregularity, as problem in
  counseling, 53
Audiovisual aids, 152

Behavioral objectives, 105
Bizarre behavior, 11
Black students, problems of, 70

Clinical evaluation, 141–161
  check lists in, 157
  feedback in, 144
  instructor reports in, 153
  minimal competency in, 143
  peer ratings in, 159
  qualification process in, 142
  self-ratings in, 159
  student progress guide in, 158
Communication, problems of, 54
Counseling, and helping relationships,
  13–28
  as base of operations, 3–12
  candidates for, 43
  definition of, 3, 8
  dual, 98
  ethical standards of, 15

Counseling (Continued)
  initiating, 11, 29
  methods of, 32
  philosophy of, 20
  principles of, 13
  reasons for, 9
  situations requiring, 10
  sources of, 24
Counseling relationship, problems in, 52
Counseling session, 29–42
  closing of, 40
  opening of, 36
  preparation for, 34
  procedure during, 38
  procedure following, 41
Counselor, characteristics of, 18
  full-time, 27
  part-time, 26
  role of, 22
Cultural differences, 70

Death, 62
Defense mechanisms, as problem in
  counseling, 53
Dependency, as problem in counseling,
  52
Depressants, in drug abuse, 48
Depression, 11
  in terminal illness, 67
Drug abuse, emergency care for, 49
  ethical aspects of, 50
  identification of, 48
  in nursing students, 45
Dying patient, 62

Educational guidance, group, 79
Educational objectives, 105
    classification of, 107
Ethics, in counseling, 15
Euthanasia, 69
Evaluation, clinical, 141–161. See also
    *Clinical evaluation.*
    measurement in, 105
Evaluation conferences, 160
Examinations, college entrance, 168. See
    also *Tests* and *Testing.*
    State Board licensure, 176

Faculty advisor, 26
Family, as counseling source, 24

Grade deficiencies, 10
Grading, in evaluation, 119
Groups, sensitivity, 86
Group counseling, 74–89
Group guidance, 74–89
    educational, 79
    vocational, 77
Guidance, definition of, 7

Hallucinogens, in drug abuse, 49
Housing, student, 210

Interviewing, 5

Learning, selection of activities in, 148
    simulated, 147
Loss of body parts, in patient, 62
Loss of function, in patient, 62

Male nurses, 58
Measurement, correlation in, 116
        definition of, 108
        normal curve in, 111
        normal distribution in, 112
        percentile scoring in, 113
        role of, 108
        scores in, 110
    in evaluation, 105–120. See also *Testing.*
    mean and standard deviation in, 114
    scales in, 109
    standardized, 117
    symbols in, 110
Men, in nursing, 58

Nurse, role of, 22, 56
Nursing schools, attrition in, 193–201

Older students, problems of, 72
Orientation programs, 75

Personality, in nursing students, studies
    of, 178, 184
Personality clash, in counseling, 53
Personnel services, for students, 216–228
    criteria for evaluation of, 216
    NLN recommendations for, 217
    Rackham Inventory of, 217

Racism, 72
Rating scales, in clinical evaluation, 155
Recommendations, student, 192
Records, and admissions, 182–192
    student, 191
Recruitment, of nursing candidates, 186
Referral, communications in, 97
    follow-up, 98
    methods of, 96
    permission for, 98
    refusal of, 97
    systems approach to, 92
Referral resources, 27, 90–100
    choice of, 92
Role playing, 147
Rules and regulations, 205

Scales, in educational measurement, 109
    rating, in clinical evaluation, 155
Schools of nursing, attrition in, 193–201
Scores, in educational measurement, 110.
        See also *Grading, Tests,* and *Testing.*
        mean and standard deviation in, 114
        percentile, 113
        standard, 115
Sensitivity groups, 86
Sensitivity training, 87
Sex education, 57
Sexuality and nursing, 57
Society, as counseling source, 24
Stimulants, in drug abuse, 49
Students, influence in counseling, 24
Student activities, 212
Student development, in nursing educa-
    tion, 202–215
Student government, 214
Student housing, 210
Student involvement, in decision making,
    209

Student personnel services, program
  evaluation, 216–228. See also *Personnel
  services.*
Student recommendations, 192
Student records, 191
Student rights, 206
  Joint Statement on, 234–240
Supervision, methods of, 149
Support, in counseling, 6


Teacher, as counseling source, 25
  role of, 22
Terminal illness, 62
Tests, achievement, 172
  American College (ACT), 168, 196
  classification type, 130
  classroom, construction of, 121–140
  College Entrance Examination Boards
    (CEEB), 168
  completion type, 124
  correction for guessing in, 132
  enumeration type, 131
  essay type, 134
  guidance, 179
  identification type, 131
  item analysis in, 133

Tests *(Continued)*
  matching type, 129
  Minnesota Multiphasic Personality In-
    ventory (MMPI), 198
  multiple-choice, 126
  objective, 124
  personality, attitude, and interest, 197
  placement, 171
  pre-entrance, 167, 195, 197
  Pre-Nursing and Guidance (PNG), 168,
    195
  situation or problem-solving, 137
  standardized, 167–181
  State Board, predicting scores in, 175
  true-false, 128
Testing, 105. See also *Measurement* and
  *Scores.*
  norm in, 118
  reliability in, 118
  validity in, 117


Vocational guidance, 77


Withdrawal behavior, 11

## DATE DUE

| | | | |
|---|---|---|---|
| NOV | | | |
| DEC 1 1982 | | | |
| | | | |
| | | | |
| | | | |
| | | | |
| | | | |
| | | | |
| | | | |
| | | | |
| | | | |
| | | | |
| | | | |
| | | | |